Cefn Coed Library

Z001686

KT-461-770

WITHDRAWN
11/06/24

PRESCRIBING IN PREGNANCY

PRESCRIBING IN PREGNANCY

Second Edition

Edited by PETER RUBIN

Professor, Department of Medicine, Queen's Medical Centre, Nottingham

BMJ
Publishing
Group

© BMJ Publishing Group 1995

All rights reserved. No part of this publication may be reproduced, stored in a retrieval system, or transmitted, in any form or by any means, electronic, mechanical, photocopying, recording and/or otherwise, without the prior written permission of the publishers.

First published in 1987

by the BMJ Publishing Group, BMA House, Tavistock Square, London WC1H 9JR

First edition 1987
Second edition 1995

British Library Cataloguing in Publication Data

A catalogue record for this book is available from the British Library

ISBN 0-7279-0949-5

Typeset by Apek Typesetters Ltd, Nailsea, Bristol
Printed and bound in Great Britain by Derry & Sons Ltd, Nottingham

Contents

Preface

The use of drugs during pregnancy and the puerperium is a question of fine balance: no harm should be allowed to befall the baby because of the drug, but equally no harm must come to the mother or baby because a disease is being inadequately treated. Information about the safe and effective use of drugs in pregnancy has not kept pace with the advances in other areas of therapeutics. Systematic research involving drugs in pregnancy is fraught with ethical, legal, and emotional difficulties, and in many cases our knowledge is based on anecdote or small studies.

The purpose of this book is to bring together what is known about prescribing in pregnancy and to put that information in a clinical context. The first edition was well received, particularly by family doctors, and this has encouraged us to produce a second edition. The chapters have all been extensively revised and updated and some have been rewritten.

I would like to thank my secretary, Louise Sabir, and Deborah Reece at the BMJ Publishing Group for their considerable help in the preparation of this book.

Peter Rubin
Nottingham
July 1995

1 General principles

PETER C RUBIN

Understanding the use of drugs during pregnancy has lagged far behind the development of knowledge in other areas of therapeutics. This is partly because "thalidomide's long shadow" has slowed research that entails giving a drug to a pregnant woman.[1] A further reason is the difficulty (often more imagined than real) in performing interdisciplinary research.

Epidemiology of drug use during pregnancy

About 35% of women in the United Kingdom take drugs at least once during pregnancy, although only 6% take a drug during the first trimester.[2] This excludes iron and vitamin supplements and drugs used during delivery. The most commonly used drugs are non-narcotic analgesics, which are taken by 12.9% of women; antibacterial agents, taken by 10.3% of women; and antacids, taken by 7.4% of women. An overview of epidemiological studies in pregnancy in North America and Europe over a 25 year period found a consistently high level of drug use.[3]

Drug use during pregnancy has decreased considerably since the last major survey in the United Kingdom in the mid-1960s. Total use has fallen from just under 80% to 35%, while the percentage of women taking self administered drugs has fallen from 64% to 9%.[4] This is probably due largely to the continued attention paid by the news media to drug induced fetal abnormality.[5]

In the puerperium the use of drugs increases substantially.[6,7] One study showed that more than 99% of women received at least one drug, often an analgesic, during the first week after delivery.[6] This study also found that hypnotics were used by 36% of women in the puerperium. There was no difference in the pattern of prescribing between mothers who were breast feeding and those who were bottle feeding.

Passage of drugs to the fetus

The placenta is essentially a lipid barrier between the maternal and fetal circulations. Drugs cross the placenta by passive diffusion. A lipid soluble, un-ionised drug of low molecular weight will cross the placenta more rapidly than a more polar drug. Given time, however, most drugs will achieve roughly equal concentrations on each side of the placenta. For example, after a single dose of indomethacin the ratio of cord to maternal plasma concentration is 0.5:1 at two hours but 1:1 at five hours.[8]

A similar example is provided by the β blockers. It was originally thought that a polar drug like atenolol might have limited transfer to the fetus, but on long term dosing this was found not to be the case.[4] Thus the practical view to take when prescribing drugs during pregnancy is that transfer of drugs to the fetus is inevitable. The only notable exceptions to this rule are heparin, insulin, and curare.

Adverse effects of drugs on the fetus and neonate

Organogenesis occurs from 18 to 55 days after conception. To have a teratogenic effect, a drug must be in the body during this critical time. A list of some commonly used drugs that are human teratogens is given in table 1.1, and the subject is covered in detail in the next chapter.

Several commonly used drugs can influence the growth or physiological function of the fetus during the period of growth and development from the end of organogenesis up to delivery.

Angiotensin converting enzyme inhibitors interere with fetal renal function by mechanisms that are not understood and produce oligohydramnios and neonatal anuria. These drugs should not be used during pregnancy.

Warfarin and *heparin* can both cause problems, one to the baby and the other to the mother. Warfarin has been associated with fetal intracranial haemorrhage, even though the maternal international normalised ratio (INR) is in the therapeutic range.

Table 1.1 Some commonly used drugs that are teratogenic in humans

Drug	Defects most commonly reported	Incidence*
Phenytoin	Craniofacial; limb	2–26%
Carbamazepine	Central nervous system; limb; cardiac	0.6–36%
Valproate	Neural tube; others?	1–2%
Warfarin	Chondrodysplasia punctata	10–25%
Retinoids†	Multiple	High
Lithium	Cardiac	<5%
Danazol	Masculinisation	Not known

* A wide range of incidence probably reflects the small size of studies and possibly selective reporting.
† Retinoids remain in the body for up to a month after the last dose of isotretinoin and two years in the case of acitretin and etretinate.

This presumably reflects differing sensitivity to warfarin between fetal and maternal tissues. Heparin can lead to osteoporosis in the mother. This has been particularly associated with doses above 15 000 units per day for more than six months.

β Blockers have about a 25% risk of causing intrauterine growth retardation when taken from early pregnancy. They do not impair growth when given only in the third trimester. The mechanism of this effect is unknown.

Tetracyclines will cause tooth discolouration, but this does not become a problem until the teeth begin to calcify at 5-6 months' gestation. There is no evidence that tetracyclines produce teratogenic effects in the first trimester.

Aspirin in analgesic doses has been shown to cause minor neonatal haemorrhage when taken within five days before delivery.

Indomethacin has been used in pregnancy both as an anti-inflammatory drug and in the treatment of preterm labour. Preterm infants exposed to indomethacin have a high incidence of adverse effects, including necrotising enterocolitis and intracranial haemorrhage. When used at the end of pregnancy indomethacin has been associated with premature closure of the ductus arteriosus.

Effect of pregnancy on drug disposition

Total body water increases by as much as 8 litres during

pregnancy,[9] and this provides a substantially increased volume within which drugs can be distributed.

Serum proteins relevant to drug binding undergo considerable changes in concentration.[10] Albumin, which binds acidic drugs such as phenytoin, decreases in concentration by up to 10 g/l.[11] The main implication of this change is in the interpretation of drug concentrations, which is discussed below.

Some liver metabolic pathways are induced during pregnancy,[12] but blood flow in the liver is unchanged.[13] Drugs with a rate of elimination that depends on the activity of liver enzymes can show large falls in serum concentration during pregnancy. That this is probably due to increased metabolic clearance is suggested by a small study of phenytoin which found clearance to be doubled during pregnancy.[14] In contrast, drugs which are eliminated at a rate mainly dependent on liver blood flow, such as propranolol, show no change in clearance during pregnancy.[15]

Renal plasma flow has almost doubled by the last trimester of pregnancy.[16] Drugs that are eliminated unchanged by the kidney are usually eliminated more rapidly. For example, the clearance of both lithium and ampicillin doubles during pregnancy.[17,18]

Therapeutic drug monitoring during pregnancy

There has been no systematic study of drug level monitoring during pregnancy and its benefits are therefore not established. However, in the case of drugs for which monitoring is readily available (anticonvulsants, lithium, and digoxin, for example) drug level monitoring can be justified on two grounds. Firstly, there is good reason to believe that the concentrations of these drugs will fall because of the physiological changes which take place during pregnancy. Secondly, compliance with drug treatment, particularly in the case of anticonvulsants, is at least as great a problem during pregnancy as at other times and if nothing else drug level monitoring will give an indication as to whether the treatment is being taken.

Two points should be considered when interpreting drug concentrations during pregnancy.

Protein binding – The reduction in albumin concentration during pregnancy leads to a decrease in the measured concentrations of drugs that are highly bound, such as

4

phenytoin. The increased amount of drug which is unbound will, however, be available for both distribution out of the blood and for elimination from the body. The net result of the change in albumin concentration on phenytoin is that the total level falls but the free level is virtually unchanged. For this reason free drug concentrations should be requested; if these are not available, the salivary levels are a good approximation.

Therapeutic range – It is not clear whether pregnancy alters the effects of drugs. This is an important matter, but it is difficult to study. Established therapeutic ranges might be inappropriate during pregnancy because of changes in the relation between drug concentration and effect.

Breast feeding

Virtually all drugs cross into breast milk. Previous dilution in the mother's body, however, coupled with the volume of milk consumed, usually means that the dose administered to the baby is clinically unimportant.

There are three main categories of drugs so far as breast feeding is concerned.

(1) Drugs that are undetectable in the baby include warfarin, which will not harm the baby if given to a nursing mother,[19] and aminoglycosides, which are not absorbed from the gastrointestinal tract of normal infants.[20]

(2) Drugs which reach the baby but in an insignificant dose include most drugs used in everyday practice: non-narcotic analgesics,[21] non-steroidal anti-inflammatory drugs,[22] penicillin and cephalosporin antibiotics,[23] antihypertensive

Table 1.2 Some commonly used drugs that should be avoided by women who are breast feeding

Amiodarone	Iodine content may cause neonatal hypothyroidism
Aspirin	Theoretical risk of Reye's syndrome
Barbiturates	Drowsiness
Benzodiazepines	Lethargy
Carbimazole	Use lowest effective dose to avoid hypothyroidism
Contraceptives (combined oral)	May diminish milk supply and reduce nitrogen and protein content
Cytotoxic drugs	Potential problems include immune suppression and neutropenia
Ephedrine	Irritability
Tetracyclines	Theoretical risk of tooth discolouration

drugs,[24] bronchodilator inhalers, and anticonvulsants (with the exception of barbiturates).[25]

(3) Drugs that reach the baby in sufficient amounts to be harmful. Some examples are shown in table 1.2, though it is important to appreciate that the adverse effects listed are often based on small numbers of case reports rather than systematic study.

Conclusion

The use of drugs during pregnancy and in the puerperium requires that a fine balance should be maintained. No harm should be allowed to befall the baby because of the drug, but equally no harm must come to the mother or baby because a disease is being inadequately treated. The aim of this book is to provide the information on which a clinical decision can be made.

1 Thalidomide's long shadow [editorial]. *BMJ* 1976; ii: 1155–6.
2 Rubin PC, Craig GS, Gavin K, Sumner D. Prospective survey of use of therapeutic drugs, alcohol, and cigarettes during pregnancy. *BMJ* 1986; 292: 81–3.
3 Bonati M, Bortolus R, Marchetti F, Romero M, Tognoni G. Drug use in pregnancy: an overview of epidemiological (drug utilization) studies. *Eur J Clin Pharmacol* 1990; 38: 325–8.
4 Forfar JO, Nelson MM. Epidemiology of drugs taken by pregnant women. *Clin Pharmacol Ther* 1973; 14: 632–42.
5 Orme ML. The Debendox saga. *BMJ* 1985; 291: 918–9.
6 Passmore CM, McElnay JC, D'Arcy PF. Drugs taken by mothers in the puerperium: inpatient survey in Northern Ireland. *BMJ* 1984; 289: 1593–6.
7 Lewis PJ, Boyland P, Bulpitt CJ. An audit of prescribing in obstetric service. *Br J Obstet Gynaecol* 1980; 87: 1043–5.
8 Traeger A, Noschel H, Zaumseil J. Zur Pharmacokinetik von Indomethazin bei Schwangeren, Kreissenden und deren Neugebornen. *Zentralb Gynakol* 1973; 95: 635–41.
9 Pirani BBK, Campbell DM, McGillivray I. Plasma volume in normal first pregnancy. *Journal of Obstetrics and Gynaecology of the British Commonwealth* 1973; 80: 884–7.
10 Studd J. The plasma proteins in pregnancy. *Clinics in Obstetrics and Gynaecology* 1975; 2: 285–300.
11 Reboud P, Groulade J, Groslambert P, Colomb M. The influence of normal pregnancy and the postpartum state on plasma proteins in lipids. *Am J Obstet Gynecol* 1963; 86: 820–8.
12 Davis M, Simmons CJ, Dordoni B, Maxwell JO, Williams R. Induction of hepatic enzymes during normal human pregnancy. *Journal of Obstetrics and Gynaecology of the British Commonwealth* 1973; 80: 690–4.
13 Munnel EW, Taylor HC. Liver blood flow in pregnancy — hepatic vein catheterisation. *J Clin Invest* 1947; 26: 952–6.
14 Lander CM, Smith MT, Chalk JB, et al. Bioavailability in pharmacokinetics of phenytoin during pregnancy. *Eur J Clin Pharmacol* 1984; 27: 105–10.
15 O'Hare MF, Kinney CD, Murnaghan JA, McDevitt DG. Pharmacokinetics of propranolol during pregnancy. *Eur J Clin Pharmacol* 1984; 27: 583–7.
16 Dunlop W. Investigations into the influence of posture on renal plasma flow and glomerular filtration rate during late pregnancy. *Br J Obstet Gynaecol* 1976; 83: 17–23.
17 Philipson A. Pharmacokinetics of ampicillin during pregnancy. *J Infect Dis* 1977; 136: 370–6.
18 Schou M, Amdisen A, Steenstrup OR. Lithium and pregnancy. II. *BMJ* 1973; iii; 137–8.

19 Orme ML, Lewis PJ, Serling MJ. Can mothers given warfarin breast feed their infants? *BMJ* 1977; i: 1564–5.
20 Milner RDG. Gentamicin in the newborn. *Postgrad Med J* 1974; **50** (suppl 7): 40–4.
21 Berlin CM, Pascuzzi MJ, Jaffe SJ. Excretion of salicylate in human milk. *J Clin Pharmacol* 1980; **27**: 245–6.
22 Needs CJ, Brooks PM. Antirheumatic medication during lactation. *Br J Rheumatol* 1985; **24**: 291–7.
23 Lipman AG. Antimicrobial agents in breast milk. *Modern Medicine* 1977; **45**: 89–90.
24 Liedholm H, Melander A, Bitzan PO, *et al.* Accumulation of atenolol and metoprolol in human breast milk. *Eur J Clin Pharmacol* 1981; **20**: 229–31.
25 Nau H, Cuhnz W, Egger HJ, Rating D, Helge H. Anticonvulsants during pregnancy and lactation. *Clin Pharmacokinet* 1982; **7**: 508–43.

2 Identifying abnormalities

KEVIN P HANRETTY, MARTIN J WHITTLE

Drugs taken during pregnancy create concern whether they are self administered or medically prescribed. The number of mothers who take drugs during pregnancy is not known, but a survey in the United States showed that about 45% of women may use at least one drug obtained by prescription and many more use drugs bought over the counter.[1] A prospective study in the United Kingdom, however, suggested that only about 10% of women took drugs in early pregnancy.[2] More recently a Finnish prospective cohort study has shown that 12% of women used analgesics during pregnancy regardless of gestation and 9% used regular medication, usually for asthma, thyroid disease, and hypertension.[3]

Defects occur in about 2% to 3% of babies at birth, of which about 25% are of genetic origin and 65% are of unknown aetiology. Only 2% to 3% of defects are thought to arise in association with drug treatment. The effect of a particular drug on the developing fetus depends on several features, including the type of agent and the gestational age at which it was taken. The aim of this chapter is to provide a guide for those involved in the care of pregnant women who have taken, or who are currently taking, drugs. Advice depends on the factors summarised in the box.

Timing of embryonic and fetal development

Several important phases in human development are recognised

Influences on the advice given to pregnant women

- Knowledge of the timing of embryonic and fetal development
- The precise nature of the teratogenic potential of the drug
- Whether the teratogenic effect is such that prenatal diagnosis is possible
- The attitude of the parents to pregnancy termination or post-natal treatment

---

(fig 2.1). During the pre-embryonic phase, from conception until 17 days (that is, about three days after the first missed period), implantation, blastocyst formation, and gastrulation take place. During this time the result of an insult to the developing organism is most likely either death and abortion (or resorption) or survival intact through multiplication of the still totipotential cells to replace those which have been lost. Embryonic development, from 18 to 55 days after conception, is when the basic steps in organogenesis occur. This is the period of maximum sensitivity since not only are tissues differentiating rapidly but damage to them becomes irreparable. The earlier in this period the insult occurs the greater the likely effect. During the fetal phase, from 56 days to term, the effects of drugs are usually limited to defects of growth and functional loss rather than gross structural abnormalities.

Drugs and their teratogenic effects

The teratogenicity of some more commonly used drugs is briefly described here.

Antibiotics

Penicillins and cephalosporins do not seem to be teratogenic.[4] In the case of antituberculous drugs, ethambutol and isoniazid have a good safety record. Streptomycin causes deafness. Rifampicin, which causes neural tube defects and facial clefting in mice, is associated with a human fetal abnormality rate two to three times higher than ethambutol or isoniazid but still within

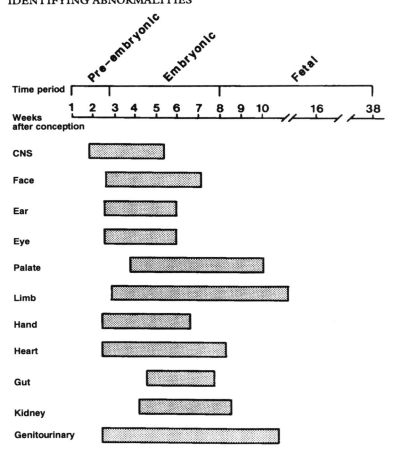

Figure 2.1 Timing of embryonic and fetal development.

the expected range. Ethionamide has been associated with exomphalos and exencephaly and should be avoided.

Psychotropic drugs

The benzodiazepines have been incriminated in the formation of oral clefts, though their teratogenicity has been disputed.[5] Tricyclic antidepressants and phenothiazines are not associated with fetal abnormality.

Lithium, which is used in the treatment of affective disorders, is associated with an increased incidence of fetal abnormality. Early data showed that it affected the cardiovascular system most often, with coarctation, patent ductus arteriosus, and mitral and tricuspid atresias being reported. The rare condition of Ebstein's anomaly, in which the tricuspid valve is distorted and displaced, occurred in a third of the affected babies, and a relative risk of between 400 and 500 was quoted.[6] More recent controlled studies have consistently shown a lower risk. The overall relative risk of fetal abnormality with lithium seems to be between 1·5 and 3·0, with a risk of cardiovascular abnormality between 1·2 and 7·7.[7] This highlights the importance of comprehensive epidemiological study of potential teratogens since adequate counselling requires accuracy.

Anticoagulants

Oral anticoagulants have been recognised as teratogens for several years[8] and are associated with three main types of abnormality.[9] Firstly, the abortion rate is increased by up to 50%, giving an overall loss rate of almost 25%. Secondly, anticoagulants can cause a well defined embryopathy, which includes shortening and stippling (chondrodysplasia punctata) of the bones and nasal hypoplasia. Both of these abnormalities occur more commonly, though not exclusively, with treatment during the first trimester. The overall incidence of the embryopathy is variously quoted and may be as high as 25%. Finally, there is a risk of serious abnormalities of the central nervous system, thought to result from dorsal midline dysplasia, which include absence of the corpus callosum, Dandy-Walker syndrome, and encephalocoeles.

Heparin may be administered in pregnancy for prophylaxis and treatment of venous thrombosis. Low molecular weight heparins seem to have practical advantages over conventional preparations. Neither type of heparin crosses the placenta.[10]

Anticonvulsants

One in 250 neonates have been exposed in utero to anticonvulsants, and a twofold to fourfold increase in the incidence of malformations has been found among the babies of epileptic mothers.[11] These include orofacial clefts and cardiac malformations (for example, septal defects), skeletal anomalies (talipes and hip dislocations), microcephaly, and neural tube defects. The phenytoin syndrome comprises craniofacial abnormalities (depressed nasal ridge, hypertelorism, clefts), limb defects (hypo-

11

plasia of distal phalanges, digital thumb, hip dislocation), and intrauterine and postnatal growth deficiencies as well as neck and rib defects and umbilical hernias.[12,13] Primidone and phenobarbitone may be teratogenic when combined with phenytoin, though the evidence for their teratogenicity when used alone is not strong. Both have been associated with facial clefting and cardiac defects.

Sodium valproate, introduced as a useful alternative to other anticonvulsants, seems to be an important teratogen and is particularly likely to produce neural tube defects, with an incidence of about 2·5%. It seems to cause spina bifida much more often than anencephaly, the ratio being 5:1 with sodium valproate compared with a normal ratio of 1·25:1 to 2·25:1. Carbamazepine also seems to be an important teratogen involved in neural tube defects and cardiovascular defects.

To prevent recurrent neural tube defect, women receiving anticonvulsant medication are strongly advised to take periconceptional folate supplements. This has reduced the incidence of recurrent neural tube defect in women with no other risk factors, but whether this result can be extrapolated to the population in question is as yet unknown.

Immunosuppressive drugs

Pregnancy in women who have undergone renal transplantation and who are taking drugs such as azathioprine and prednisolone is becoming increasingly common. Studies in patients with ulcerative colitis and Crohn's disease show little evidence that either of these drugs is teratogenic in humans.[14]

Cyclosporin has been implicated in some central nervous system anomalies, but evidence is scanty.

Sex hormones

Hormone preparations taken in early pregnancy include the oral contraceptive pill and those used in threatened abortion. Despite numerous studies, the teratogenic effects of sex hormones remain uncertain. Three main groups of abnormalities may occur: limb reductions; cardiac defects, especially transposition of the great vessels; and central nervous system defects such as hydrocephaly and neural tube lesions. The constellation of disorders termed VACTERAL (vertebral, anal atresia, cardiac, tracheo-oesophageal atresia, and renal and limb defects) has in some studies been significantly associated with ingestion of hormones in early pregnancy.[15]

The relative risk of cardiovascular abnormality is increased in women who take hormone preparations. A recent review based on a reanalysis of data from the US Collaborative Perinatal Study, a large prospective study of fetuses exposed to female sex hormones between the first and fourth months of gestation, showed that this increase is in the order of 2·48.[16]

Most studies did not distinguish between oral contraceptives and progestagens used for threatened abortion or, in the past, determining pregnancy. This distinction is clearly of great practical importance. It seems unlikely, but has not definitely been proved, that oral contraceptives are teratogenic.

Women receiving treatment for anovulatory infertility may be exposed to gonadotrophin releasing hormone agonists in early pregnancy. There are few current data, but initial studies are reassuring.[17]

Dermatological preparations

The introduction of retinoids as effective agents for severe acne, a condition that affects women in the reproductive age group, has led to a new spectrum of teratogenesis. Teratogenic effects are seen in up to 25% of babies born to mothers who took retinoids, with as many again affected by mental retardation. The role of these compounds has recently been reviewed,[18] but the most important issue relating to etretinate is that it can cause teratogenesis for up to two years after treatment has stopped. All the main systems have been affected, including craniofacial, cardiac, and central nervous system disorders, and the spontaneous abortion rate is increased.

Management of pregnancy and potential teratogenesis

Teratogenesis concerns two main groups of patients: women already taking drugs for a chronic underlying illness and those who have taken a single course of treatment, unaware of an early pregnancy. Women in the former group should be counselled before their pregnancy so that they are fully aware of the risks of teratogenesis and how to reduce the chance of fetal malformation. Such an approach demands close cooperation between physicians,

13

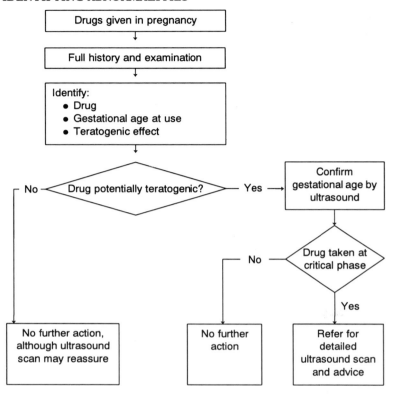

Figure 2.2 Action to be taken when a patient may have used drugs in pregnancy.

general practitioners, and the prenatal diagnosis team. As, all too often, the patient first presents in pregnancy, we suggest the following scheme, which aims to establish accurately the gestational age at the time of exposure to the drugs and the potential for prenatal diagnosis (fig 2.2).

History

Menstruation – A careful record of the recent dates of periods and the menstrual cycle should always be sought. Gestational age is more likely to be correct if the first day of the last period has been noted and the preceding cycles were regular (every 28 days), although even then up to 15% of calculations will be wrong by 14 days or more.

Conception – It is always worth inquiring whether the woman knows when conception occurred; occasionally, remarkably accurate calculations are made.

Treatment – Once the gestational age has been established, the exact time of exposure to the drugs must be determined. This may require a review of the patient's notes either from the general practitioner or the hospital. Careful identification of the drugs taken is vital, not just by the group – "I think it was something for my nerves" – but by name. The possibility that more than one drug was taken should also be considered. The patient may forget to mention the most important drug, and taking several drugs together may result in a higher incidence of teratogenesis. Patients should also be asked about self medication, as they may report only medically prescribed preparations.

Investigation – Accurate estimation of gestational age is essential. Although a good history will help, dating by ultrasound scanning using fetal crown-rump length in the first trimester or, between 12 and 20 weeks, the biparietal diameter, should allow the dates to be calculated to within about a week. With these data the exact stage in pregnancy at which treatment was given can be established. Quite often it can be shown that the mother was not pregnant at the time of exposure or had passed the time at which teratogenesis would be likely to occur.

Prenatal diagnosis

If drugs were taken at a critical gestational age the most effective method of excluding fetal anomaly is by high resolution ultrasound scanning. The advent of transvaginal ultrasound has made it possible to diagnose certain abnormalities, including anencephaly, in the first trimester.[19] In later pregnancy transabdominal ultrasound provides extraordinarily good images of the fetal brain and spine; the heart; the arms, legs, and hands; and the face (fig 2.3).

Fetal anomalies associated with teratogens may be broadly grouped into defects of the central nervous system, cardiovascular system, arms and legs, facial clefting, and multisystem defects. Most structural anomalies should be detectable by about 20 to 22 weeks, although this depends on several different factors; it is impossible to provide exact rates of detection.

Central nervous system – One of the commonest indications for ultrasound examination in pregnancy is to exclude neural tube

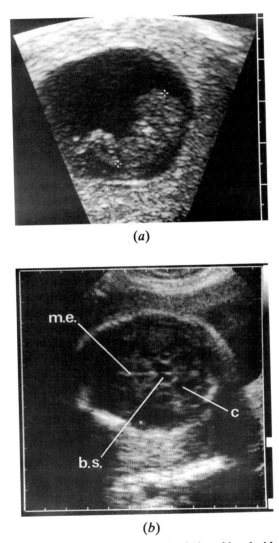

(a)

(b)

Figure 2.3 Ultrasound scans. (a) This shows the clarity achieved with transvaginal scanning of a 10 week fetus. (b) Fetal brain (m.e. = midline echo, b.s. = brain stem, c = cerebellum). (c) Longitudinal view showing fetal spine. (d) Four chamber view of fetal heart (f.o. = foramen ovale, l.v. = left ventricle, r.v. = left ventricle, i.v.c. = intraventricular septum). (e) Fetal long bones, (fi = fibula, t = tibia, f = foot). (f) Fetal hand (h = hand, t = thumb).

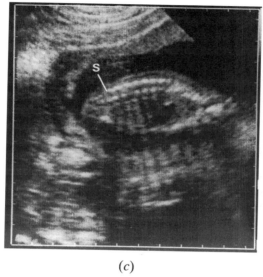

(c)

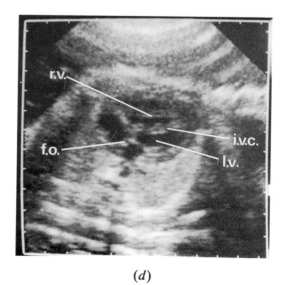

(d)

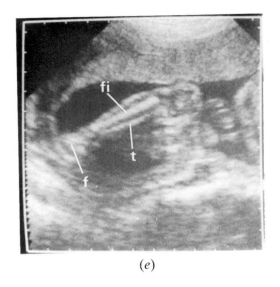

(*e*)

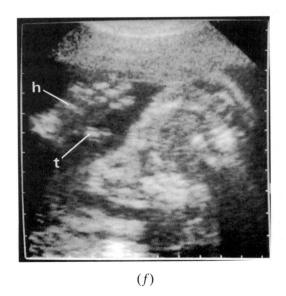

(*f*)

defects. Anencephaly can usually be identified about 12 weeks after the last period, but spina bifida is more subtle and is best detected at 16 to 18 weeks. The predictive ability of ultrasound examination depends on good equipment, a high level of training, good fetal position, and the mother not being excessively obese. In one series of neural tube defects all cases of anencephaly were detected, as well as 96 of 102 cases of spina bifida. In two cases spina bifida was wrongly diagnosed.[20] The value of measuring maternal serum α fetoprotein concentration and performing amniocentesis is debatable in patients already referred for a detailed scan, when a lesion would be unlikely to be missed. If fetal views are poor, however, amniocentesis would be indicated in the presence of increased serum α fetoprotein concentration. The high incidence of spina bifida in the babies of women taking anticonvulsants would certainly indicate the need for amniocentesis if views were unsatisfactory.[21]

Cardiovascular system – Fetal cardiology is a relatively recent development, reflecting the vast improvements in the quality of imaging. Most serious heart defects, particularly those of connections, should be detectable by 18 to 20 weeks. The basic requirement in cardiac scanning is to obtain a four chamber view, which if normal will exclude many important abnormalities. Effort should also be directed at obtaining views of the great vessel connections. Gross defects, such as Ebstein's complex, will have been detected by scan.[22]

Deformities of the arms and legs – Although it is relatively easy to measure the fetal limbs, abnormalities of growth may not become apparent until later in pregnancy. Gross deformities of the type associated with thalidomide should, however, be detected by 18 weeks. Abnormalities of the hands and even equinus deformities of the feet may be seen in optimal conditions.

Facial clefting – This seems to be a common feature of teratogenesis, and although it is not usually in itself an indication for terminating pregnancy, the display of normality may be some comfort to anxious parents.

Multiple anomalies – This group of anomalies can often be detected early in pregnancy and usually by 16 weeks. In the VACTERAL complex, features of the arms, legs, kidneys, and heart should be detectable by 18 to 20 weeks. Vertebral defects may be seen earlier, but tracheo-oesophageal fistula and anal atresia may not be diagnosed until delivery.

Conclusions

The exact role of drugs in producing fetal abnormalities remains uncertain, and some apparently unexplained fetal anomalies may be the result of a forgotten toxic insult. In general terms we recommend the formation of a team, comprising a clinical pharmacologist and members of a prenatal diagnostic unit, which could provide rapid and effective advice.

Key points

- The time of maximum teratogenic potential is 18–55 days after conception: tissues are differentiating rapidly and damage is irreparable

- Retinoids are high grade teratogens which can exert their effect up to two years after the last dose

---

1 Schardein JL. Current status of drugs as teratogens in man. *Prog Clin Biol Res* 1985; 163C: 147–53.
2 Rubin PC, Craig GF, Gavin K, Sumner D. Prospective study of use of therapeutic drugs, alcohol, and cigarettes during pregnancy. *BMJ* 1986; 292: 81–3.
3 Heikkila AM, Erkkola RU, Nummi SE. Use of medication during pregnancy - a cohort study on use and policy of prescribing. *Annales Chirurgiae et Gynaecologiae* 1994; 83 (suppl 208): 80–3.
4 Greenberg G, Inman WHW, Weatherall JAC, Adelstein AN, Haskey JC. Maternal drug histories and congenital abnormalities. *BMJ* 1977; ii: 853–6.
5 Weber LWD. Benzodiazepines in pregnancy–academic debate or teratogenic risk. *Int J Biol Res Pregnancy* 1985; 6: 151–67.
6 Linden S, Rich CL. The use of lithium during pregnancy and lactation. *J Clin Psychiatry* 1983; 44: 358–61.
7 Cohen LS, Friedman JM, Jefferson JW, Johnson EM, Weiner ML. A re-evaluation of risk of in utero exposure to lithium. *JAMA* 1994; 271: 146–50.
8 Bloofield DK. Fetal deaths and malformations associated with the use of coumarin derivatives in pregnancy. *Am J Obstet Gynecol* 1980; 107: 883–8.
9 Hall JG, Pauli RM, Wilson KM. Maternal and fetal sequelae of anticoagulation during pregnancy. *Am J Med* 1980; 68: 122–40.
10 Fejgin MD, Lourwood DL. Low molecular weight heparins and their use in obstetrics and gynecology. *Obs Gyn Survey* 1994; 49: 424–31.
11 Lindhout D, Omtzigt JGC. Teratogenic effects of antiepileptic drugs: implications for the management of epilepsy in women of childbearing age. *Epilepsia* 1994; 35 (suppl 4): S19–28.
12 Kelly TD. Teratogenicity of anticoagulant drugs: review of the literature. *Am J Med Genet* 1984; 19: 413–34.
13 Albengres E, Tillement JP. Phenytoin in pregnancy: a review of the reported risks. *Int J Biol Res Pregnancy* 1983; 4: 71–4.

14 Witter FR, King TM, Blake DA. The effects of chronic gastrointestinal medication on the fetus and neonate. *Obstet Gynecol* 1980; **58**: 798–848.

15 Schardein JL. Congenital anomalies and hormones during pregnancy. A clinical review. *Teratology* 1980; **22**: 251–70.

16 Hook EB. Cardiovascular birth defects and prenatal exposure to female sex hormones: a re-evaluation of data re-analysis from a large prospective study. *Teratology* 1994; **49**: 162–6.

17 Wilshire GB, Emmi AM, Gagliardi CC, Weiss G. Gonadotropin-releasing hormone agonist administration in early human pregnancy is associated with normal outcomes. *Fertil Steril* 1993; **60**: 980–3.

18 Geiger JM, Baudin M, Saurat JH. Teratogenic risk with etretinate and acitretin treatment. *Dermatology* 1994; **189**: 109–16.

19 Cullen MT, Green J, Whetham J, et al. Transvaginal ultrasonographic detection of congenital abnormalities in the first trimester. *Am J Obstet Gynecol* 1990; **163**: 466.

20 Campbell S, Smith P, Pearce JM. The ultrasound diagnosis of neural tube defects and other craniospinal abnormalities. In: Rodeck CH, Nicolaides KH, eds. *Prenatal diagnosis. Proceedings of the 11th study group of the Royal College of Obstetricians and Gynaecologists.* London: RCOG 1983: 245–57.

21 Weinbaum PJ, Cassidy SB, Vintzileos AM, Campbell WA, Ciarleglio L, Nochimson DJ. Prenatal detection of a neural tube defect after fetal exposure to valproic acid. *Obstet Gynecol* 1986; **67**: 31–3.

22 Allan LD, Desai G, Tynan MJ. Prenatal echocardiographic screening for Ebstein's anomaly for mothers on lithium therapy. *Lancet* 1983; **ii**: 875–6.

3 Treatment of common minor ailments

COLIN W HOWDEN

A number of common minor disorders may occur in pregnancy and require drug treatment for control of symptoms. These include headache and musculoskeletal pains as well as a variety of gastrointestinal complaints, including heartburn, nausea, vomiting, dyspepsia, and constipation. This chapter reviews the drugs used to treat such complaints with respect to efficacy and safety and appraises the available evidence in an attempt to recommend the safest drugs.

Use of analgesics

Simple analgesics are the commonest drugs taken in pregnancy and are self administered. Aspirin, paracetamol, ibuprofen, and a variety of analgesic combinations are available in Britain without prescription. Many women consume analgesics in the early stages of pregnancy before realising they are pregnant. Collecting and interpreting controlled data on exposure to analgesics and the incidence of congenital defects is therefore difficult.

Aspirin

Evidence linking ingestion of aspirin to fetal malformations is suggestive but inconclusive. Massive doses of aspirin given to pregnant rats cause congenital skeletal and eye defects.[1] Many of the studies suggesting a teratogenic effect of aspirin in humans have been retrospective case-control studies. For example, among 833 women who had given birth to malformed babies there was a higher incidence of ingestion of aspirin during early pregnancy than in a control group.[2] In a large prospective cohort study of more than 50 000 women, however, no increase in congenital abnormalities was found in the babies of mothers who had taken aspirin during pregnancy when compared with control patients who had not taken aspirin.[3]

Aspirin has been thought to cause a reduction in birth weight and an increase in the stillbirth rate.[4] In a prospective cohort study of more than 41 000 women, however, the stillbirth rate was 1·4% both in women who consumed large quantities of aspirin and those who took no aspirin during pregnancy.[5] Similarly, the neontal death rate was 1·1% in both groups.

Aspirin is freely transferable across the placenta and is excreted by the newborn infant at a slower rate than in adults owing to immaturity of the excretory pathways. The infant of a woman who ingested regular therapeutic doses of aspirin throughout pregnancy took five days to eliminate the drug.[6]

One potential problem of aspirin in newborn infants is its effect on haemostatic mechanisms. In a case-control study haemostasis was normal in 33 of 34 pairs of mothers and infants where there was no history of aspirin ingestion.[7] There were, however, abnormalities of platelet adhesiveness in most of the infants whose mothers had taken aspirin within five days of delivery. There was also a higher incidence of minor bleeding in the babies whose mothers had taken aspirin. Furthermore, intrapartum blood loss from the mothers was greater in those who had recently taken aspirin.

The use of low dose aspirin during pregnancy may be increasing,[8] given its possible beneficial effects in preventing pregnancy-induced hypertension and intrauterine growth retardation. In a small Italian study, no haemorrhagic complications were noted in 10 newborn babies of mothers who had taken 50 mg aspirin daily from week 12 of gestation.[9] Serum thromboxane concentrations in the babies were reduced immediately after birth but returned to normal by day 4. Low dose aspirin does not seem to have any adverse effects on the development of the fetal cardiovascular system.[10]

Paracetamol

The effects of paracetamol during pregnancy have not been studied as extensively as those of aspirin, but it seems to be generally safe. Studies in animals have shown no adverse effects on fetal or placental growth.[11] There is nothing to suggest that paracetamol in normal dosage is associated with any specific problems during pregnancy or breast feeding, and it is recommended as the mild analgesic of choice.[12]

Treatment of nausea and vomiting

Although common in early pregnancy, nausea and vomiting are generally of short duration and can often be managed without drugs. Women should be reassured and advised to take small frequent meals and to avoid large amounts of fluid. Drug treatment is often necessary, however, if symptoms are severe or prolonged.

Antiemetic drugs have been linked to a number of congenital defects. One large prospective series showed an association between vomiting in early pregnancy and certain congenital abnormalities, but no correlation could be established with any specific antiemetic drug.[13] This led to the proposal that it was vomiting rather than antimetic treatment which was causally associated with birth defects. In a prospective study of more than 16 000 women, however, there was no difference in the incidence of congenital defects between those who had vomited in pregnancy and those who had not.[14] The authors concluded that any increased risk in women taking antiemetic drugs was related to the drugs rather than the vomiting and that the risk was low in any case. Specific drugs are considered below.

Debendox

Debendox, a combination of dicyclomine, doxylamine, and pyridoxine, was highly successful in the management of nausea and vomiting during pregnancy. Sporadic case reports linking its use to congenital abnormalities caused concern, however, about its safety in pregnancy. This highlights the problems about drawing conclusions from uncontrolled data since both retrospective[15,16] and prospective[17,18] studies did not confirm any teratogenic effect. In the United States, the Food and Drug Administration also concluded that there was no firm evidence linking this preparation with birth defects.[19] Nevertheless, the manufacturers withdrew the drug in 1983 because of the unsubstantiated claims about teratogenicity.[16]

24

Antihistamines

Antihistamines are generally recommended for treating nausea and vomiting in pregnancy but often don't work.[20–22] Meclozine and cyclizine are widely used and seem to be safe. Concern about an association between the use of these drugs and congenital malformations, particularly cleft palate, has not been substantiated in prospective controlled studies.[23,24] There may, however, be a weak association between meclozine and congenital eye defects.[24] Promethazine may be associated with an increased incidence of congenital dislocation of the hips.[13,25]

Metoclopramide

Data on the effects of metoclopramide on early fetal development are lacking. It has been used in late pregnancy and in the management of hyperemesis gravidarum.[26] Since it increases lower oesophageal sphincter pressure and accelerates gastric emptying metoclopramide has been used in labour and before anaesthesia,[27] when it is considered safe and efficacious. The combination of metoclopramide and omeprazole has been studied for the prevention of gastric aspiration in obstetrical anaesthesia.[28] Oral omeprazole with parenteral metoclopramide was generally successful in reducing gastric juice acidity and volume before anaesthesia.

Non-pharmacological approaches

Recently, there have been some preliminary small controlled studies looking at alternative approaches to managing the nausea and vomiting of pregnancy. Sensory affect stimulation was compared with placebo in a crossover study in 23 women within the first 14 weeks of pregnancy and improved the symptoms in 87%, compared with 43% who were given placebo.[29] Self administered acupressure was compared with "sham" acupressure in a controlled study in 60 women.[30] Symptoms improved in both groups, but there was a significantly greater improvement in nausea in patients treated with acupressure. However, no difference in the frequency of vomiting was seen. Assuming that the efficacy of this sort of approach can be verified in further randomised, placebo controlled, blinded studies, and that these treatments can be made acceptable to patients, such non-pharmacological treatment could be important in the future.

25

Treatment of heartburn and dyspepsia

Heartburn due to gastro-oesophageal reflux is extremely common during pregnancy, particularly in the second and third trimesters. Lower oesophageal sphincter pressure is reduced throughout pregnancy and is lowest around the 36th week.[31]

Patients with symptoms of reflux should be reassured and advised to take small, frequent meals rich in carbohydrates and to avoid stooping or lying flat. If drug treatment is necessary, teratogenicity is a less important issue because most cases start in late pregnancy. Non-absorbable antacids such as aluminium hydroxide or magnesium trisilicate may be used, although aluminium antacids given alone may cause constipation. Antacids are safe when taken in the second or third trimester, although they have been associated with an increased rate of congenital defects when taken in early pregnancy.[22]

Dyspepsia that is not related to oesophageal reflux is unusual in pregnancy. In particular, peptic ulcer rarely presents for the first time during pregnancy. In women with existing peptic ulcer, symptoms tend to improve as the pregnancy progresses, but some may still require treatment. Simple measures include cessation of smoking, small regular meals, and antacids for relief of symptoms.

The H2-receptor antagonists are safe and effective for managing peptic ulcer in non-obstetric practice. Routine use in pregnancy cannot, however, be recommended because of the lack of appropriate data on their safety. H2-antagonists have been successfully used before general anaesthesia for caesarean section to reduce gastric acidity and prevent aspiration of acid into the lungs (Mendelson's syndrome). Both cimetidine and ranitidine are excreted into breast milk, but there are no data to suggest a harmful effect on the baby.

Sucralfate has not been widely used during pregnancy in the United Kingdom, but it is an effective treatment for peptic ulcer and has been recommended for use in pregnancy in the United States because it is not absorbed.[32] It is now understood that most peptic ulcers are a result of chronic inflammation induced by infection with *Helicobacter pylori*. Eradication of this infection has been recommended for all ulcer patients.[33] However, this treatment approach has not been studied in pregnancy and cannot be recommended. Compounds containing bismuth should be avoided; the effects on fetal development of the absorption of small quantities of bismuth are unknown.

In summary, dyspepsia in pregnancy, whether related to peptic ulceration or not, is probably best managed with reassurance, advice on meals and smoking, and non-systemic antacids.

Treatment of constipation

Patients should be advised to take a diet high in cereal fibre and fresh fruit. Simple constipation is best treated by a bulking agent such as preparations containing bran, ispaghula, or methylcellulose. Stimulant laxatives may be uterotonic and are therefore contraindicated during pregnancy.

Conclusions

It is a counsel of perfection that no drugs should be used in pregnancy, but some minor symptoms of common ailments often require treatment for the comfort of the mother. Paracetamol seems to be the safest minor analgesic; an antihistamine compound can probably be safely prescribed for a short period for treating nausea and vomiting; and heartburn and dyspepsia are best managed along simple lines, with an antacid in early pregnancy and possibly metoclopramide in the later stages.

Key points

- Paracetamol is the mild analgesic of choice during pregnancy
- Drug treatment of nausea and vomiting is often unrewarding; antihistamines are probably the best of a fairly ineffective range of options
- Simple antacids are safe when taken in the second or third trimesters for the treatment of heartburn and dyspepsia
- Avoid stimulant laxatives as they may stimulate the uterus

---

1 Warkany J, Takacs E. Experimental productions of congenital malformation in rats by salicylate poisoning. *Am J Pathol* 1959; 35: 315–31.
2 Richards JD. Congenital malformations and environmental influences in pregnancy. *Br J Prev Soc Med* 1969; 23: 218–25.
3 Slone D, Siskind V, Heinonen OP. Aspirin and congenital malformations. *Lancet* 1976; i: 1373–5.

4 Turner G, Collins E. Foetal effects of regular salicylate ingestion in pregnancy. *Lancet* 1975; ii: 338–9.
5 Shapiro S, Siskind V, Monson RR. Perinatal mortality and birth-weight in relation to aspirin taken during pregnancy. *Lancet* 1976; i: 1375–6.
6 Garrettson LK, Procknal JA, Levy G. Fetal acquisition and neonatal elimination of a large amount of salicylate. Study of a neonate whose mother regularly took therapeutic doses of aspirin during pregnancy. *Clin Pharmacol Ther* 1975; 17: 98–103.
7 Stuart MJ, Gross SJ, Elrad H, Graeber JE. Effects of acetylsalicylic-acid ingestion on maternal and neonatal hemostasis. *N Engl J Med* 1982; 307: 909–12.
8 Bremer HA, Wallenburg HC. Low dose aspirin in pregnancy: Changes in patterns of prescribing in the Netherlands. *Eur J Obstet Gynecol Reprod Biol* 1993; 52: 29–33.
9 Valcamoncio A, Foschini M, Soregaroli M, Tarantini M, Frusco T. Low dose aspirin in pregnancy - a clinical and biochemical study of the effects in the newborn. *J Perinat Med* 1993; 21: 235–40.
10 Veille JC, Hanson R, Sivakiff M, Swain M, Henderson L. Effects of maternal ingestion of low-dose aspirin on the fetal cardiovascular system. *Am J Obstet Gynecol* 1993; 168: 1430–7.
11 Lubawy WC, Burris-Garrett RJ. Effects of aspirin and acetaminophen on fetal and placental growth in rats. *J Pharm Sci* 1977; 66: 111–3.
12 De Swiet M. *Medical disorders in obstetric practice.* Oxford: Blackwell Scientific, 1984.
13 Kullander S, Kallen B. A prospective study of drugs and pregnancy. II. Antiemetics. *Acta Obstet Gynecol Scand* 1976; 55: 105–11.
14 Klebanoff MA, Mills JL. Is vomiting during pregnancy teratogenic? *BMJ* 1986; 292: 724–6.
15 Harron DWG, Griffiths K, Shanks RG. Debendox and congenital malformations in Northern Ireland. *BMJ* 1980; 281: 1379–81.
16 Zierler S, Ruthman KJ. Congenital heart disease in relation to maternal use of Benedictin and other drugs in early pregnancy. *N Engl J Med* 1985; 313: 347–52.
17 Milkovich LM, Van der Berg BJ. An evaluation of the teratogenicity of certain antinauseant drugs. *Am J Obstet Gynecol* 1976; 125: 244–8.
18 Smithells RW, Sheppard S. Teratogenicity testing in humans: a method of demonstrating safety of Benedictin. *Teratology* 1978; 17: 31.
19 Food and Safety Administration. *Federal Register* 1979; 44: 41068.
20 Lewis PJ, Chamberlain GVP. Treatment of everyday complaints in pregnancy. *Prescribers' Journal* 1982; 22: 77–84.
21 Fagan EA, Chadwick VS. Drug treatment of gastrointestinal disorders in pregnancy. In: Lewis PJ, ed. *Clinical pharmacology in obstetrics.* Bristol: Wright, 1983: 114–37.
22 Nelson MM, Forfar JO. Associations between drugs administered during pregnancy and congenital abnormalities of the foetus. *BMJ* 1971; i: 523–7.
23 Smithells RW, Chinn ER. Melclozine and foetal malformation: a prospective study. *BMJ* 1964; i: 217–8.
24 Shapiro S, Kauffman DW, Rosenberg L. Melclozine in pregnancy in relation to congenital malformations. *BMJ* 1978; i: 487.
25 Huff PS. Safety of drug therapy for nausea and vomiting of pregnancy. *J Fam Pract* 1980; 11: 969–70.
26 Singh MS, Lean TH. The use of metoclopramide in hyperemeisis gravidarum. *Proceedings of the Obstetrics and Gynecology Society of Singapore* 1970; i: 43.
27 Howard FA, Sharp DS. Effect of metoclopramide on gastric emptying in labour. *BMJ* 1973; i: 446–8.
28 Orr DA, Bill KM, Gillon KR, Wilson CM, Fogarty DJ, Moore J. Effects of omeprazole with and without metoclopramide in elective obstetric anaesthesia. *Anaesthesia* 1993; 48: 114–9.
29 Evans AT, Samuels SN, Marshall C, Bertolucci LE. Suppression of pregnancy-induced nausea and vomiting with sensory affect stimulation (SAS). *J Reprod Med* 1993; 38: 603–6.
30 Belluomini J, Litt RC, Lee KA, Katz M. Acupressure for nausea and vomiting of pregnancy: a randomized controlled study. *Obstet Gynecol* 1994; 84: 245–8.
31 Van Thiel DH, Gavaler JS, Joshi SN, Stremple J. Heartburn of pregnancy. *Gastroenterology* 1977; 72: 666–8.
32 Lewis JH, Weingold AB. The use of gastrointestinal drugs during pregnancy and lactation. *Am J Gastroenterol* 1985; 80: 912–21.
33 NIH Consensus Development Panel. *Helicobacter pylori* in peptic ulcer disease. *JAMA* 1994; 272: 65–9.

4 Antibiotics

RICHARD WISE

Young women often develop infections, particularly of the urinary tract, and pregnant women commonly require antimicrobial treatment. Their urine should be cultured at the first antenatal visit – ideally in the first trimester. Bacteriuria occurs in about 5% of pregnancies (as many as 15% in some racial groups) and if it is not treated between a quarter and a third of patients may develop pyelonephritis, with consequent danger to their own health and an increased incidence of fetal loss.[1]

Because pregnant women are often in an environment with young children they are at greater risk of developing the more trivial upper respiratory infections, which may require treatment. Occasionally, they need treatment for more serious infections. It is therefore necessary to know which antimicrobial agents can be used with negligible risk for the minor infections and to have some appreciation of the balance of risks for more serious cases.

In assessing the risk to the fetus several points should be considered. For many antimicrobial agents we now have more than 30 years' experience of freedom from congenital abnormality. Many studies have been performed in animals; though these are important, their results should be viewed with some reservation. For example, sulphonamides can cause gross fetal malformations when given in high doses to mice and rats,[2] but 50 years of use would surely have shown a teratogenic propensity in humans, and this, to my knowledge, has not been recorded. One of the reasons why laboratory animals make poor models for studying fetal damage is the profound effect of large doses of antimicrobial agents on the animal's gastrointestinal flora and consequently on the animal's metabolism.

On the other hand, certain drugs should definitely be avoided.

For example, streptomycin causes neonatal ototoxicity after long term treatment of maternal tuberculosis.[3,4] It follows, by implication rather than by hard information, that the other aminoglycosides, such as gentamicin, tobramycin, netilmicin, and amikacin, should be avoided for minor infections. In the treatment of serious maternal infection, however, the undoubted efficacy of these drugs should be balanced against the theoretical risks.

Pregnant and non-pregnant women differ considerably in the way in which they handle antimicrobial agents, and this may influence treatment. Philipson showed that serum concentrations of ampicillin in women who were 9–36 weeks pregnant were half the values found in the same women when they were not pregnant.[5] Low maternal concentrations have been described after dosage with most antimicrobial agents, including aminoglycosides. The therapeutic implications of these low concentrations are difficult to assess. Failure of antibiotic treatment might incorrectly be blamed on the wrong choice of antibiotic, and the drug might be replaced by a potentially more toxic agent. This could be particularly dangerous when treating a serious infection with an agent such as an aminoglycoside, when the natural caution of the doctor against giving what he or she might consider to be high doses will in fact cause more problems.

In general, full adult doses should be used when treating infections in pregnant women. When serious infections are to be treated with an aminoglycoside, for example, assays should be performed to ensure that the patient is receiving sufficient drug and that neither she nor the fetus is being exposed to unacceptably high levels. Similarly, the length of treatment should be dictated by the disease and not be influenced unduly by the fact that the patient is pregnant. Inadequate treatment, which may be followed by further courses of antibiotics, is likely to put mother and fetus at greater risk than a full course of the correct antimicrobial agent.

In recent years the length of a course of antibiotic therapy has been generally shortened. In bacteriuria in pregnancy a 7–14 day course of treatment was usually prescribed, but now investigations suggest a single dose[6,7] or high dose short course[8]; perhaps a reasonable approach is to prescribe an initial 3 day course with an appropriate agent and if bacteriuria returns a further 3 day course followed by prophylactic 50 mg nitrofurantoin each night until the puerperium.[9] These patients should then be investigated for a urinary tract abnormality.

Antimicrobial agents

Table 4.1 lists various antimicrobial agents together with their possible toxic effects on the fetus in early or late pregnancy, and a safety rating. "Probably safe" indicates that no significant risk to the fetus has been documented and hence such agents constitute a first choice if an antimicrobial agent has to be used; "caution" indicates that effects on the fetus have been recorded with the agent (or a chemically related compound) or that its mode of action suggests a theoretical risk, but there may well be times when the balance of risks suggests that such compounds should be used. "Avoid" indicates that the agent carries a definite risk and its use might imply negligence (unless there was an overwhelming reason to the contrary). Such division of the compounds is obviously somewhat subjective.

Treatment of common conditions

Table 4.2 lists some of the common infections likely to be encountered in pregnancy. The first choice of treatment is usually an agent listed as probably safe in table 4.1, although not necessarily so. A second choice agent might have to be used if the patient is allergic to a first choice compound or the bacteria responsible are resistant to the first choice agent. In this context it is particularly important to take cultures from pregnant patients before treatment so that a safe and efficacious change can be made to treatment if the patient does not respond or the causative organism proves resistant to initial treatment. The clinician should eschew the temptation to use too low a dose. If the infection needs treating at all it needs full dosage.

Urinary tract infection

The most common reason for pregnant women to take antibiotics is for acute cystitis or covert bacteriuria. The choice of treatment is between ampicillin (or its close relative amoxycillin) and cephalexin (as the oral cephalosporin with which there is more experience). Cephalexin is probably more suitable because about half the common Gram negative bacteria which cause urinary tract infections are resistant to ampicillin. Although a combination of amoxycillin and clavulanic acid (Augmentin) has been used in pregnancy and it would overcome the problem of resistance, this combination might best be reserved

Table 4.1 Antimicrobial agents and their possible adverse effects

		Adverse effects on fetus		
Agent	Use	First trimester	Second and third trimester	Comments
Penicillin (benzylpenicillin and phenoxymethylpenicillin)	Probably safe		Allergy; possibility of sensitising the fetus	All the commoner β-lactams may be described as safe
Long acting penicillins	Probably safe		Allergy; possibility of sensitising the fetus	Little information available but no suggestion of increased toxicity
Ampicillin	Probably safe		Allergy; possibility of sensitising the fetus	
Ampicillin prodrugs: talampicillin, pivampicillin, bacampicillin				Little information available. Reasonable to avoid prodrug formulation and use the parent ampicillin
Amoxycillin	Probably safe		Allergy; possibility of sensitising the fetus	
Amoxycillin and clavulanic acid (Augmentin)	Probably safe		Allergy; possibility of sensitising the fetus	Little information available. Best avoid until more experience reported
Antipseudomonal penicillins: carbenicillin, mezlocillin, azlocillin, ticarcillin, piperacillin	Probably safe		Allergy; possibility of sensitising the fetus	Little information available. Reserve for treatment of serious infections caused by susceptible bacteria
Antistaphylococcal penicillins: flucloxacillin and cloxacillin	Probably safe		Allergy; possibility of sensitising the fetus	
Oral cephalosporins: cephalexin, cefaclior, cephradine	Probably safe		Allergy; possibility of sensitising the fetus	Little information available especially on newer introductions (cefixime, cefpodoxime)

Injectable cephalosporins:	Probably safe	Allergy; possibility of sensitising the fetus	Little information. These agents are probably safe and might well be reasonable choices in treatment of severe infection. Agents containing N-methylthiotetrazole side chain should be avoided on theoretical grounds – that is, interference with vitamin K metabolism (cefamandole in the UK)
Sulphonamides: All agents	Probably safe in first trimester; avoid within 2 days of delivery	Avoid (within two days of delivery); kernicterus	Risk is greater for more highly protein bound agents, such as sulphafurazole, rather than sulphamethoxazole
Trimethoprim	Probably safe		Theoretical teratogenic risk of folic acid antagonist. Risk of megaloblastic anaemia preventable by folinic acid
Co-trimoxazole (trimethoprim and sulphamethoxazole)	Probably safe (but see sulphonamide above)	Kernicterus	Considerable experience of safety in first trimester
Tetracyclines: all agents	Avoid	Discoloration and dysplasia of teeth and bones; cataracts	Possible hepatotoxicity in mother
Aminoglycosides: Streptomycin	Avoid	Ototoxicity	Little reason to be used. A better choice can be made in tuberculosis and serious sepsis

continued overleaf

33

Table 4.1 *continued*

Agent	Use	Adverse effects on fetus		Comments
		First trimester	Second and third trimester	
Gentamicin, tobramycin, netilmicin, amikacin	Caution		Theoretical risk of ototoxicity suggested	Effective in serious sepsis; regular assay required
Spectinomycin	Probably safe			Reserve for treatment of gonorrhoea when penicillin resistance or allergy is a problem
Fusidic acid	Probably safe			Wide experience suggests safety.
Quinoloines: nalidixic acid	Caution			Deposition in growing bones in certain animals and in the teeth of young children. Interferes with bacterial DNA; theoretical risk to humans
Recently developed drugs: ciprofloxacin, norfloxacin, enoxacin, ofloxacin, pefloxacin	Avoid			No experience in pregnancy – see nalidixic acid
Nitrofurantoin	Probably safe			Theoretical risk of haemolysis in glucose-6-phosphate dehydrogenase deficiency. Prophylactic use
Vancomycin, teicoplanin	Caution			Safety data not available in humans. Reserve for treatment of serious staphylococcal sepsis
Macrolides and lincosamides: Erythromycin base stearate	Probably safe			
Erythromycin estolate	Avoid			Maternal hepatotoxicity in late pregnancy

Clarithromycin, azithromycin, Lincomycin and clindamycin	Avoid		Maternal pseudomembranous colitis. Avoid unless no other suitable agents available
Metronidazole	Caution	Theoretical risk of teratogenesis	No evidence of teratogenicity in humans. Benefit will probably outweigh risk in serious anaerobic sepsis
Chloramphenicol	Avoid	Grey baby syndrome	Little evidence of ill effect to fetus in early pregnancy. Remember possible maternal blod dyscrasias. Usually a safer choice can be made
Antituberculosis agents: Rifampicin	Caution	Postnatal bleeding	Avoid in mothers with liver disease. High dosage teratogenicity in animals. Benefits probably outweigh risks. Vitamin K should be given to mother and neonate
Isoniazid	Probably safe		
Ethambutol	Probably safe		Observe mother for jaundice
Para-aminosalicylic acid	Probably safe		Now little used
Pyrazinamide	Caution		Little information available
Antifungal agents: Amphotericin	Caution		Limited information; safety not established
Flucytosine	Avoid	Teratogenic in animals	
Ketoconazole, fluconazole	Caution		Limited information; safety not established
Miconazole	Caution		
Griseofulvin	Avoid	Teratogenic in animals	
Nystatin (topical)	Probably safe		Absorbed from vaginal topical use

continued overleaf

Table 4.1 *continued*

Agent	Use	Adverse effects on fetus		Comments
		First trimester	Second and third trimester	
Antimalarial drugs:				
Chloroquine	Probably safe			Safety established in low dose, except for rare reports of hearing loss in children
Quinine	Avoid	Possible abortifacient		
Proguanil	Probably safe			
Pyrimethamine and dapsone (Maloprim)	Avoid			Teratogenicity reported in rats, but no convincing evidence in humans. Maloprim and Fansidar have been associated with fatalities
Pyrimethamine and sulphadoxine (Fansidar)	Avoid			
Primaquine	Avoid			
Antiparasitic agents:				
Piperazine	Probably safe			
Mebendazole	Avoid	Possible teratogenic		
Thiabendazole	Caution			Safety not established
Praziquantrel	Caution			Safety not established
Antiviral agents:				
Amantadine	Avoid	Embryotoxic in animals		Unless there is a life threatening infection in the mother it is probably best to avoid antiviral agents in pregnancy

36

Acyclovir	Probably safe, but use only when potential benefits outweigh risk	Theoretical risk. Acts as "chain terminator"
Vidarabine	Avoid	Teratogenic in animals
Zidovudine	Not currently licenced in pregnancy	Little evidence of teratogenicity
		Evidence of reduced vertical transmission of HIV

Table 4.2 Common infectious conditions in pregnancy and recommended treatment

Condition	First choice treatment	Second choice treatment	Comments
Asymptomatic bacteriuria or simple cystitis	Ampicillin, amoxycillin (if isolate sensitive) or cephalexin by mouth	Nitrofurantoin, sulphonamide, or trimethoprim (or co-trimoxazole)	In asymptomatic bacteriuria treatment should probably last 7–10 days. Simple acute cystitis may respond to a single dose or short course
Acute pyelonephritis	Cefuroxime, ampicillin intravenously (if isolate sensitive)	Gentamicin intravenously	
Pharyngitis	Benzylpenicillin intravenously, procaine penicillin intramuscularly, or phenoxymethylpenicillin by mouth	Erythromycin base	Note: 70–80% of cases of pharyngitis are caused by viruses
Bronchitis	Ampicillin by mouth or amoxycillin	Erythromycin	
Lobar pneumonia	Benzylpenicillin	Erythromycin	If not pneumococcal, change in treatment may be required
Legionnaires' disease	Erythromycin plus rifampicin		
Endocarditis prophylaxis	Amoxycillin by mouth	Erythromycin	Follow recommendations of working party[9]
Endocarditis treatment:			
Streptococcal	Benzylpenicillin + gentamicin		
Staphylococcal	Flucloxacillin + fusidic acid	Vancomycin	
Gonorrhoea	Benzylpenicillin intramuscularly	Cefuroxime or spectinomycin	Spectinomycin if patient is β-lactam allergic
Infection caused by Chlamydia trachomatis	Erythromycin by mouth		Erythromycin should be given for 7–10 days

Prophylaxis for abdominal operations:			
Gastric or biliary	1 dose cefazolin	1 dose co-trimoxazole	
Appendicectomy or colonic	1–3 doses amoxycillin and clavulanic acid (Augmentin)	1–3 doses gentamicin plus metronidazole	
Tuberculosis	Rifampicin + isoniazid + ethambutol		Rifampicin and isoniazid should be given for 9 months and ethambutol for 3 months. Pyridoxine supplements should be given with isoniazid
Malarial prophylaxis	Chloroquine		See text
Serious undiagnosed sepsis	Gentamicin intravenously plus anti-pseudomonal penicillin intravenously, possibly plus metronidazole	Broad spectrum cephalosporin intravenously (such as cefuroxime or ceftazidime)	On establishing causative pathogen it may be possible to omit gentamicin if organisms are susceptible to antipseudomonal penicillin and the patient has made a satisfactory response

for difficult cases until more evidence about its safety has accumulated. Women who are allergic to β lactams can be given a short course of trimethoprim, preferably alone or with sulphamethoxazole in the first, and probably the second, trimester; in the third trimester nitrofurantoin would be an acceptable alternative.

Pharyngitis and tonsillitis

Most sore throats are caused by viruses and are therefore not susceptible to treatment. Patients with signs of systemic infection such as tachycardia, fever, and enlarged cervical lymph nodes should be given penicillin. If the infection is severe this should be given parenterally followed by phenoxymethylpenicillin. Patients allergic to penicillin should receive erythromycin base.

Bronchial and pulmonary infections

An acute bacterial bronchial infection after a viral bronchitis is not uncommon in a previously healthy young woman. The first choice of treatment is either ampicillin or amoxycillin. A specimen for culture should be taken, however, because 10–20% of *Haemophilus influenzae* are resistant to these two drugs. If the patient fails to respond this might be a reasonable indication for a course of treatment with a combination of amoxycillin and clavulanic acid.

The commonest cause of lobar pneumonia in a previously well young woman is *Streptococcus pneumoniae*, and this should be treated with benzylpenicillin or with erythromycin if the patient is allergic to benzylpenicillin. Legionnaires' disease is a common cause of community acquired pneumonia. There is still some doubt about the best treatment for this condition, but present knowledge suggests erythromycin. In seriously ill patients rifampicin may be added; however, this agent does not have a licence in the United Kingdom for legionella infections.

Surgical prophylaxis

Although elective operations are avoided in pregnancy, emergency operations may be necessary. The same guidelines for the choice of the correct prophylactic antibiotic should be followed – namely, that a short course of an appropriate agent should be given. If there is no evidence of established intra-abdominal sepsis (such as an appendix abscess) one to three doses of a parenteral cephalosporin such as cefuroxime plus metronidazole should be given (or possibly amoxycillin and clavulanic acid alone). If an abscess has formed then three to four days' treatment is required after drainage.

Septicaemia

Happily, it is rare to have to treat a pregnant patient who has possible septicaemia that has not been diagnosed microbiologically. In septicaemia the risks to the patient outweigh the risks to the fetus and broad spectrum antimicrobial agents in full dosage should be prescribed. Parenteral cefuroxime would be a good first choice, possibly with the addition of metronidazole if there is evidence of intra-abdominal sepsis. Once a pathogen and its antimicrobial susceptibilities have been determined, treatment can be directed at that organism.

Tuberculosis

Because of the chronic nature of tuberculosis it is not uncommon to encounter this infection in pregnancy. Young women who are not pregnant should be warned of the increased risk of failure of the contraceptive pill if, as is likely, rifampicin is prescribed.

Opinions differ on the treatment of infections with *Mycobacteria tuberculosis* in pregnant women. This difference is mainly concerned with the risks associated with rifampicin, which readily crosses the placenta; teratogenicity has been suggested but not confirmed. Treatment should not be appreciably different from that in non-pregnant patients and should be of full duration. Streptomycin is rarely used in tuberculosis and should certainly be avoided in pregnant women. Treatment by a physician who specialises in respiratory medicine is advisable.

Malaria prophylaxis and treatment

Malaria is an important cause of abortion, premature labour, and perinatal death, as well as affecting the mother. Hence both prophylaxis and treatment are required during pregnancy. Prophylaxis should be started one week before visiting a malarial area and continued for one month after leaving. For travel to north Africa and the Middle East, where chloroquine resistance has not been reported, chloroquine 300 mg weekly is advised. Travel to a country where chloroquine resistant *Plasmodium falciparum* is found presents a problem. Pyrimethamine and sulfadoxine (Fansidar) and pyrimethamine and dapsone (Maloprim) are now considered to carry sufficient risk of Stevens-Johnson syndrome and neutropenia respectively to almost outweigh their benefits, not only in pregnant women but in any individual. Pregnant women should be advised not to visit an area where chloroquine resistant *P falciparum* is found (such as east and central Africa, South East Asia, and South America). For women who intend to visit a major urban centre only (where the risk is smaller) chloroquine 300 mg a week plus proguanil 200 mg a day should be prescribed.

In the treatment of benign malaria (caused by *P vivax, P ovale,* and *P malariae*) chloroquine should be used; radical cure with primaquine should not be undertaken until after pregnancy to avoid the possibility of haemolysis due to glucose-6-phosphate dehydrogenase deficiency. *P falciparum* malaria should be treated with chloroquine unless the patient comes from an area where chloroquine resistance is known. In such cases quinine should be used. Quinine will reduce the numbers of parasites in the blood and after a three day course a single dose of three tablets of Fansidar is warranted. Then, if asexual parasites are still present in a blood smear a seven day course of erythromycin should be given.

Other parasitic infections

Toxoplasmosis – Fetal infection in the first trimester is relatively uncommon, but in most of the cases that do occur the disease is severe. In the last trimester, however, infection of the fetus by an infected mother is more usual, but most babies will have no overt disease at birth. The treatment suggested is pyrimethamine 50 mg twice weekly, plus folic acid 5 mg daily, plus sulphadiazine 50 mg/kg twice daily. Patients should have treatment for two weeks, followed by four weeks without treatment; this should be repeated throughout pregnancy. Spiramycin may also have a role in this disease. Anyone considering treating a patient with possible toxoplasmosis should liaise with an expert in this disease.

Amoebiasis – Metronidazole 800 mg three times daily should be given for five days, followed by diloxanide furonate 500 mg three times daily for five days (to eliminate trophozoites from the gut lumen).

Giardiasis – Metronidazole 400 mg three times daily should be given for seven days. Relapses are not uncommon.

Helminthiasis – Most infections with ascaris and trichuris are asymptomatic and are best left alone in pregnancy. Occasionally, a 4 g dose of piperazine may be required. Heavy hookworm infections should be treated with 5 g of bephenium or 10 mg/kg of prantel pamoate if anaemia is severe.

Venereal diseases

As penicillin forms the basis of the treatment of both gonorrhoea and syphilis there is no need for any change in treatment in pregnancy, and both conditions should be treated vigorously and followed up (in both mother and infant). Penicillin resistant gonococci should be treated with an injectable cephalosporin.

A problem can arise in the treatment of syphilis in pregnant women who are allergic to penicillin. It is doubtful if erythromycin is satisfactory in eradicating spirochaetes from the fetus. In such cases it might be reasonable to use tetracycline because the effect of congenital syphilis on the teeth (not to mention other sites) would be more severe than the effect of tetracycline. Chlamydial infections causing non-specific urethritis during pregnancy should be treated with erythromycin.

Pelvic inflammatory disease

Pelvic inflammatory disease is not uncommon in pregnancy and treatment is difficult. Patients should be given erythromycin together with metronidazole (except in the first trimester).

Antibiotics and lactation

Both mother and general practitioner are often anxious that antimicrobial agents being used to treat the mother are being transferred to the infant. Although most antibiotics are found in breast milk in low concentrations, they are unlikely to affect the child. This is because appreciable amounts of the agent will not be absorbed from the infant's gastrointestinal tract – for example, the aminoglycosides and injectable cephalosporins – or, if the agents are absorbed, the concentrations reached in the infant are extremely low – for example, ampicillins. Concern has been expressed, however, over a few agents.

Chloramphenicol – Although grey baby syndrome is most

unlikely (as concentrations are too low), the possibility of infant marrow toxicity necessitates either avoiding this agent or stopping breast feeding.

Tetracyclines – Tetracyclines should be avoided because of the theoretical, rather than real, risk of teeth discolouration. Chelation of the tetracycline by the calcium ions in milk probably overcomes this problem.

Sulphonamides (including co-trimoxazole) – Although the risk of kernicterus is low, it should be borne in mind especially if a highly protein bound sulphonamide – for example, sulphadimethoxine – is being used. In glucose-6-phosphate dehydrogenase deficiency there is the risk of haemolytic anaemia.

Isoniazid – There is a theoretical risk of convulsions with isoniazid. Both mother and baby should be given pyridoxine.

Metronidazole – Mothers who start taking metronidazole after they have started breast feeding may find that it has an adverse effect on the taste of the milk.

Conclusion

A wide range of antimicrobial agents is now available and harmful effects on the fetus have been proved for relatively few. Infection in pregnant women usually requires treatment and the choice of agent should not be a major problem.

Key points

- Harmful effects on the fetus have been proved for relatively few antimicrobial agents
- Full adult doses should generally be used to treat infections in pregnant women
- The length of treatment should be dictated by the disease and not influenced unduly by the fact that the patient is pregnant
- Even though they are found in breast milk in low concentrations, antibiotics are unlikely to affect the child

---

1 Condie AP, Brumfitt W, Reeves DS, Williams JD. The effects of bacteriuria in pregnancy on foetal health. In: Brumfitt W, Asscher AW, eds. *Urinary tract infection*. London: Oxford University Press, 1973:108–16.

2 Kato T, Kitagawa S. Production of congenital abnormalities in fetuses of rats and mice with various sulphonamides. *Congenital Abnormalities* 1973; 13: 7–15.

3 Assael BM, Parini R, Rusconi F. Ototoxicity of aminoglycoside antibiotics in infants and children. *Pediatr Infect Dis* 1982; 1: 357–67.

4 Conway N, Birt BD. Streptomycin in pregnancy: effect on the foetal ear. *BMJ* 1965; ii: 260–3.

5 Philipson A. Pharmacokinetics of antibiotics in pregnancy and labour. *Clin Pharmacokinet* 1979; 4: 297–309.

6 Harris RE, Gilstrap LC, Pretty A. Single dose antimicrobial therapy for asymptomatic bacteriuria during pregnancy. *Obstet Gynecol* 1982; 59: 546.

7 Bailey RR, Bishop V, Reddie BA. Comparison of single dose with a 5 day course of co-trimoxazole for asymptomatic (covert) bacteriuria in pregnancy. *Aust NZ J Obstet Gynaecol* 1983; 23: 41.

8 Anderstan KJ, Abbas AMA, Davey A, Ancill RJ. High dose, short course amoxycillin in the treatment of bacteriuria in pregnancy. *Br J Clin Prac* 1983; 37: 212–4.

9 Bailey RR. Management of uncomplicated urinary tract infections. *Internat J Antimicrob Chemother* 1994; 4: 95–100.

10 Working Party of the British Society for Antimicrobial Chemotherapy. The antibiotic prophylaxis of endocarditis. *Lancet* 1982; ii: 1323–6.

5 Treatment of Asthma

CATHERINE NELSON-PIERCY,
JOHN MOORE-GILLON

At least 3% of women of child bearing age have some degree of asthma,[1] and this prevalence is increasing. Asthma is by far the most common chronic illness of young adulthood, and all those involved in the care of women during pregnancy and childbirth will encounter asthmatic patients. This chapter outlines the normal physiological changes in the respiratory system during pregnancy and the interactions between asthma and pregnancy, and goes on to deal with the special considerations relating to prescribing for pregnant women with asthma.

Changes in respiratory function during pregnancy

During pregnancy, oxygen consumption is increased by around 20% and the maternal metabolic rate by about 15%. This extra demand is met by a 40–50% increase in resting minute ventilation, resulting mainly from a rise in tidal volume rather than respiratory rate. This change in ventilation may be due to the respiratory stimulant effect of progesterone. The maternal hyperventilation leads to a reduction in partial pressure of arterial carbon dioxide to 4·0 kPa, and there is a compensatory fall in serum bicarbonate concentration to 18–22 mmol/l. A mild respiratory alkalosis is therefore normal in pregnancy, with an arterial pH of 7·44.

Up to three quarters of women feel breathless at some time during pregnancy, possibly because of an increased awareness of the physiological hyperventilation. This "dyspnoea of pregnancy"

46

is most common in the third trimester and may lead to diagnostic confusion.

Late in pregnancy the diaphragmatic elevation caused by the enlarging uterus leads to a decrease in functional residual capacity, but diaphragm excursion is unaffected so vital capacity is unchanged.

The effect of pregnancy on asthma

Published evidence about the effect of pregnancy on asthma is conflicting, and there is no consistent trend to improvement or worsening of disease severity.[2] Most studies investigating the course of asthma in pregnancy have been too small to draw valid conclusions, although a review of more than 1000 pregnant women with asthma reported in nine studies found a worsening of asthma in 22%, improvement in 29%, and no change in 49%.[3]

In general, the course of asthma in pregnancy in individual patients is unpredictable. There may be some relation to the severity of asthma before pregnancy in that women with only mild disease are unlikely to experience problems, whereas those with severe asthma are at greater risk of deterioration, particularly late in pregnancy.[3,4] Those women whose symptoms improve during the last trimester of pregnancy may experience postnatal deterioration.[4,5]

Whatever happens to the severity of the disease process itself, many asthmatic patients experience worsening of their symptoms during pregnancy simply because they have stopped or reduced their usual medication due to fears (their own or those of their doctors) about its safety.

Effect of asthma on pregnancy and its outcome

In most women, asthma has no effect on the outcome of pregnancy. Severe, poorly controlled asthma, however, may have an adverse effect on fetal outcome.[6] This is thought to be the result of chronic or intermittent maternal hypoxaemia. Early studies suggested a slight increase in the risk of premature labour,[6–8] and this has been confirmed.[9,10] A large prospective American study of 3891 deliveries found an association between maternal asthma and preterm labour (relative risk = 2·33, 95% confidence interval 1·03 to 5·26),[11] and the retrospective study of

Perlow and colleagues similarly showed that preterm delivery occurred significantly more often in asthmatic women than controls.[12]

There is also some evidence of an association between asthma and babies of low birth weight.[3,11,12] The influence is small but seems to be related to the effectiveness of asthma control.

Some studies have reported an increased incidence of pregnancy induced hypertension or pre-eclampsia in asthmatic women.[6,13,14] In over 24 000 women without essential hypertension, Lehrer and colleagues found a significant association between pregnancy induced hypertension and asthma during pregnancy.[13] These studies need to be interpreted with caution: women with asthma are likely to be seen more frequently during the antenatal period than normal women, and therefore to have their blood pressure measured more often. The more frequent the measurements, the more likely it is that transient increases in blood pressure will be discovered.

Recent studies suggest an increased incidence of transient tachypnoea of the newborn,[15] neonatal hypoglycaemia,[14] neonatal seizures,[16] and admission to the neonatal intensive care unit[10] in the babies of asthmatic women, but the magnitude of effect on any adverse perinatal outcome is certainly small and related to the degree of control of the asthma.

In conclusion, it seems that there may be a slight increased risk to the babies of asthmatic mothers, but this risk is small and may be minimised by maintaining good control of asthma throughout pregnancy.

Management of asthma in pregnancy

Much unnecessary impairment of quality of life results from failure to diagnose or adequately treat asthma. Since virtually all women are under some form of medical supervision during pregnancy, this is an ideal time to recognise previously undiagnosed asthma and to achieve optimum disease control in women known to be asthmatic.[17]

The successful management of asthma during pregnancy requires a cooperative approach between the obstetrician, the physician managing the asthma, and the woman. The aim of treatment is to achieve virtual total freedom from symptoms, such that the life style of the individual is not affected. The past 10 or so years have seen major changes in approaches to asthma management. The emphasis now is on the prevention, rather than the treatment, of acute attacks. Regular inhaled anti-inflammatory medication is now considered first line maintenance treatment for all but those with infrequent symptoms (less than once a day).[18] There is also now a greater focus on home peak flow monitoring and personalised self management plans, which have been shown to reduce morbidity in patients with asthma.[19,20]

The drug treatment of asthma in pregnancy is, in essence, no different from the treatment of asthma in non-pregnant women. All the drugs in widespread use to treat asthma, including systemic steroids, seem to be safe. Considerations concerning individual treatments are discussed below.

Corticosteroids

Systemic corticosteroids have serious and well known side effects when given frequently or in high doses for prolonged periods. Women and their doctors are accordingly reluctant to use these drugs in pregnancy, and their concern extends to the use of inhaled corticosteroids. This concern is misplaced, and steroids should be used to treat asthma in pregnancy in the same way and for the same reasons as outside pregnancy.

Short courses of oral steroids are required for exacerbations of asthma that fail to respond to an increased dose of inhaled steroids, and for acute severe attacks. Rarely, a patient with severe asthma may require long term maintenance oral steroids. Such individuals will always also take inhaled steroids to minimise the oral dose requirement and risk the usual side effects of systemic steroids.

Other than media-fed concern about drugs falling within the broad category of "steroids," there is a single 40 year old report of an increased incidence of cleft palate in the offspring of rabbits treated with cortisone early in gestation.[21] This finding has never been reproduced in humans despite the fact that steroids have been used extensively during pregnancy for a variety of conditions. Prednisolone is metabolised by the placenta and very little (10%) active drug reaches the fetus. There is no evidence of increased risk of abortion, stillbirth, congenital malformations, adverse fetal effects, or neonatal death attributable to treating the mother with steroids.[7,8,22]

Although suppression of the fetal hypothalamic-pituitary-adrenal axis is a theoretical possibility when the mother is treated with systemic steroids, there is no evidence from clinical practice to support this. Further reassurance comes from a study in which the adrenocortical reserve of six newborns whose mothers had received long term systemic steroids was formally assessed – the response to exogenous adrenocorticotrophic hormone was normal.[23] Maternal adrenal insufficiency is, however, a possibility, and if the woman has been taking more than 7·5 mg of prednisolone for two weeks or more, parenteral steroids (hydrocortisone 100 mg three or four times a day) should be given to cover the stress of labour and delivery.

Prolonged use of oral steroids increases the risk of gestational diabetes and causes a deterioration in blood glucose control in those women with established impairment of glucose tolerance in pregnancy. Provided clinicians are aware of this and check the blood glucose concentration regularly, the hyperglycaemia is amenable to treatment with diet and, if required, insulin, and is reversible on stopping or reducing the steroid dose. The development of hyperglycaemia is not, however, an indication to discontinue or decrease the dose of oral steroids, the requirement for which must be determined by the asthma.

Few women with asthma will be taking oral steroids; most will be receiving inhaled steroids. As with systemic steroids, no harm to the fetus from inhaled steroids has been shown. Furthermore, only minimal amounts of inhaled corticosteroid preparations are systemically absorbed.[24] This should be emphasised, as decreasing or stopping treatment with inhaled anti-inflammatory drugs during pregnancy often causes potentially dangerous deterioration in disease control.

Beclomethasone dipropionate is the oldest inhaled steroid preparation, and therefore the drug for which most information exists. Several studies have shown no increased incidence of congenital malformations or adverse fetal effects attributable to the use of inhaled beclomethasone in pregnancy.[8,25,26] There is less information about the more recently introduced inhaled steroid budesonide, but it is widely used and seems safe. Use of a spacer device with inhaled steroids will reduce oropharyngeal candidiasis, improve delivery of the drug, and decrease the possibility of systemic effects. Fluticasone proprionate is a newer inhaled corticosteroid, and even though there is no evidence of hazard it is sensible to use a more long established alternative if possible.

In summary, inhaled, oral, and parenteral corticosteroids are safe in pregnancy. The addition of systemic corticosteroids to control exacerbations of asthma is appropriate, and these must not be withheld if current medications are inadequate.

β sympathomimetics (β₂ agonists)

Inhaled β agonists such as salbutamol and terbutaline provide rapid and effective relief of bronchospasm in most patients. Tremor and tachycardia are the most common dose related side effects of these drugs, but they occur far less commonly than with the now little used oral preparations. In patients with impaired glucose tolerance, pulmonary oedema, hypokalaemia, and hyperglycaemia are potential but rare adverse effects when high doses of β_2 agonists are given intravenously (to treat acute severe asthma or preterm labour).

Transfer of β_2 agonists from the systemic circulation across the placenta is relatively rapid,[27] but very little of a given inhaled dose reaches the lungs and only a minute fraction of this reaches the systemic circulation. A recent prospective study of 259 pregnant women with asthma treated with inhaled β_2 agonists showed no difference in perinatal mortality, congenital malformations, birth weight, Apgar scores, or delivery complications in comparison with asthmatic women not using β agonists and non-asthmatic controls.[28] There has been concern that β agonists may delay the onset of labour or cause prolonged labour, but there is no evidence that this occurs with inhaled preparations.

The inhaled, long acting β_2 agonist salmeterol may be used in some patients who have not achieved adequate control of symptoms with regular inhaled corticosteroids and short acting β_2 stimulants. Salmeterol is especially useful for those with nocturnal asthma.[29] Its safety in pregnancy has not yet been adequately established.

Disodium cromoglycate and nedocromil

Inhaled cromoglycate is more widely used in the management of asthma in children than adults. It seems to be safe for both mother and fetus. A French study of nearly 300 pregnant women showed no increased risk of malformations,[30] and there have been no suggestions of other ill effects in over 30 years of use.

Nedocromil is a more recently introduced preparation with a pharmacological action similar to that of sodium cromoglycate. There are no reports of adverse effects on the fetus, but insufficient data exist to support its routine use in pregnancy.

Methylxanthines

Methylxanthines are no longer used as first line therapy for asthma. A modified release oral preparation may be added to conventional treatment with inhaled bronchodilators and inhaled corticosteroids, especially to control night time symptoms in certain patients.[31] Both theophylline and aminophylline readily cross the placenta, and fetal theophylline concentrations are similar to those of the mother.[32] Although theophylline has been shown to be a cardiovascular teratogen in animals, there is no conclusive evidence of ill effect of malformation in the human fetus.[33,34] One recent report links theophylline with congenital cardiac anomalies in human,[35] but the drug has been used extensively over a period of decades and is widely regarded as safe.

Pharmacokinetic data concerning xanthines in pregnancy are conflicting. The increased blood volume associated with pregnancy may lead to lower concentrations of active drug. In contrast, a small study suggested a 20–35% reduction of theophylline clearance in the third trimester,[36] but this has not been confirmed by more recent studies.[37,38] Some have noted transient tachycardia or irritability in neonates of mothers receiving xanthines, but others found mean neonatal heart rate and Apgar scores were unaffected by maternal use of theophylline.[32]

Anticholinergic drugs

Anticholinergic drugs have traditionally been considered more effective in the management of chronic bronchitis than asthma, but inhaled ipratropium bromide may be worth trying when symptoms are not optimally controlled with regular inhaled corticosteroids and β_2 agonists. No adverse fetal effects have been reported but, as with atropine, there is a minimal increase in fetal heart rate.

Management of acute severe asthma

Acute severe attacks of asthma are dangerous and should be vigorously managed in hospital. The treatment is no different from the emergency management of acute severe asthma in non-pregnant patients. Oxygen, nebulised bronchodilators, oral or intravenous steroids, and, in severe cases, intravenous aminophylline or intravenous β_2 agonists should be used as indicated. Sudden severe deterioration, or failure to respond to treatment, should raise the possibility of a pneumothorax. The ionising radiation from chest radiography is approximately 0·2 rads (less than 1/20th of the maximum recommended exposure (5 rads) in pregnancy, and abdominal shielding will minimise the exposure to the fetus. If a chest radiograph is clinically indicated this investigation must not be withheld just because the patient is pregnant.

Other considerations when prescribing for pregnant women with asthma

Education and reassurance of asthmatic women before conception as well as during pregnancy are integral parts of management. This should ensure that women do not discontinue, reduce, or withhold vital medication just because they are pregnant. Women with asthma may justifiably be reassured about the outlook for themselves and their baby during pregnancy.

Aspirin

Low dose aspirin is gaining acceptance as prophylaxis for certain women at very high risk of early onset pre-eclampsia,[39] but it is worth remembering that some asthmatic patients may develop severe bronchospasm with aspirin, and pregnant asthmatic women should be asked about a history of such sensitivity before being treated with low dose aspirin.

Management of respiratory infection

Upper and lower respiratory tract infections, bacterial and viral, are common precipitants for deterioration in asthma symptoms. The production of yellow or green phlegm is not pathognomonic of a bacterial lower respiratory tract infection and may just indicate an exacerbation of asthma with eosinophils in the sputum. However, if there are other pointers to infection (fever for example), antibiotics should be prescribed.

The antibiotics most frequently used in respiratory infections, including the penicillins, cephalosporins, and erythromycin, are safe in pregnancy. Amoxycillin should be given in higher than usual dosage (500 mg 8 hourly) in pregnancy because of increased renal clearance. Tetracycline causes permanent staining of the child's teeth, has adverse effects on the fetal skeleton, and is contraindicated in pregnancy, with rare exceptions where the health of the mother takes precedence over the risk to the fetus. Similarly, cough medicines containing iodine are contraindicated since the iodine is taken up by the fetal thyroid and may cause hypothyroidism and fetal goitre.

Adults in general, and pregnant women in particular, are susceptible to varicella zoster (chicken pox) pneumonia, and the maternal and fetal mortality is high.[40] Because of the substantial risk to the mother, non-immune pregnant women exposed to varicella should be given zoster immune globulin.[41] Patients taking systemic corticosteroids are at especially high risk of severe varicella, and it has recently been suggested that patients should be asked about a history of varicella before starting to take steroids.[42] If the history is doubtful, antibody status should be checked; those who are seronegative must be told that they should attend immediately and receive prophylaxis with zoster immune globulin if they are inadvertently exposed to varicella. The risk of varicella is particularly relevant for the few pregnant women with asthma who need systemic corticosteroids.

Management during labour and delivery

Although they are one of the most common fears of asthmatic women entering pregnancy, acute attacks of asthma during labour and delivery are extremely rare, and women should be reassured accordingly. The explanation for this rarity is uncertain, although it is possible that it is related to an increase in endogenous corticosteroid or catecholamine production at this time. Neither of the two indirect deaths attributed to asthma in the recent confidential inquiry into maternal deaths in the UK occurred during labour.[43] Women should continue with their regular inhalers throughout labour, and those receiving maintenance oral steroids (> 7·5 mg prednisolone daily) or being treated with steroids for more than two weeks before the onset of labour or delivery should receive parenteral steroids during labour and until they are able to restart their oral medication.

If prostaglandin is used to induce labour, to ripen the cervix, or for early termination of pregnancy, prostaglandin $F_{2\alpha}$ should be avoided as it may cause bronchospasm.[44,45] Prostaglandin E_2 is a bronchodilator and is safe to use.

All forms of pain relief in labour, including epidural analgesia and Entonox, may be safely used by asthmatic women, although in the unlikely event of an acute asthmatic attack opiates should be avoided. If anaesthesia is required, women should be encouraged to have epidural rather than general anaesthesia because of the increased risk in people with asthma or chest infection and associated atelectasis. Although ergometrine has been reported to cause bronchospasm, particularly in association with general anaesthesia, this does not seem to be a practical problem when Syntometrine (oxytocin/ergometrine) is used to prevent post-partum haemorrhage.

Breast feeding

Women with asthma should be encouraged to breast feed their babies if they wish. The risk of atopic disease developing in the child of an asthmatic woman is about 1 in 10, or 1 in 3 if both parents are atopic. There is some evidence that this risk may be reduced by breast feeding. A 15 year prospective study has shown that breast feeding and delaying exposure to allergens reduces the frequency of clinical allergic disease,[46] and prolonged breast feeding may lower the incidence of severe or obvious atopic disease, particularly in babies with a family history of atopy.[47]

All the drugs used to manage asthma, including oral steroids, are safe to use when breast feeding. Small amounts of prednisone and prednisolone are secreted in breast milk,[48,49] and although continuous maternal use of high doses of corticosteroids could theoretically affect the infant's adrenal function, this is unlikely with doses below 30 mg prednisolone per day. No clinical side effects have been reported in infants breast fed by mothers receiving prednisolone. A small study examining the secretion of tritium labelled prednisolone in breast milk showed that a mean of only 0·14% of radioactivity from an oral dose of 5 mg of prednisolone was recovered per litre of breast milk.[48]

Theophylline appears in breast milk, with a milk to plasma ratio of 0·7, reaching a peak concentration two hours after peak plasma concentrations.[50] We are not aware of any reports of important problems in clinical practice resulting from transfer of methylxanthines in breast milk, and the proportion of new mothers whose asthma cannot be well controlled without the use of methylxanthines is in any case extremely small.

Conclusion

Management of asthma in pregnancy does not differ significantly from management outside pregnancy. The priority should be effective control of the disease process, with the aim being total freedom from symptoms both day and night. Great attention must, however, be given to explanation and reassurance about the safety, in pregnancy and during lactation, of the drugs used to treat asthma.

The small risk of harm to the fetus comes from poorly controlled severe asthma rather than from the drugs used to prevent or treat asthma. Good control of asthma reduces the already small risks of preterm delivery or low birth weight. Furthermore, it sets a pattern for future management; the mother-infant relationship may not flourish in the presence of chronic maternal ill health. Asthma in pregnancy should accordingly be regarded as an opportunity to gain long term benefit, not just as a challenge lasting nine months.

Key points

- Many asthmatic women get worse in pregnancy because they stop taking their medication

- Regular inhaled anti-inflammatory medication is first line maintenance treatment

- The drug treatment of asthma in pregnancy is the same as in non-pregnant women

- Steroids should be used to treat asthma in pregnancy if clinically indicated; there is no evidence that they are harmful to the fetus

- If chest radiography is clinically indicated then it should be performed

---

1 Littlejohn PI, Ebrahim S, Anderson R. Prevalence and diagnosis of chronic respiratory symptoms in adults. *BMJ* 1989; **298**: 1556–60.
2 Sims CD, Chamberlain GVP, de Swiet M. Lung function tests in bronchial asthma during and after pregnancy. *Br J Obstet Gynaecol* 1976; **83**: 434–7.
3 Gluck JC, Gluck P. The effects of pregnancy on asthma: a prospective study. *Ann Allergy* 1976; **37**: 164–8.
4 White RJ, Coutts I, Gibbs CJ, MacIntyre C. A prospective study of asthma during pregnancy and the puerperium. *Respir Med* 1989; **83**: 103–6.
5 Juniper EF, Daniel EE, Roberts RS, Kline PA, Hargreave FE, Newhouse MT. Improvement in airway responsiveness and asthma severity during pregnancy. A prospective study. *Am Rev Resp Dis* 1989; **140**: 924–31.
6 Bahna SL, Bjerkedal T. The course and outcome of pregnancy in women with bronchial asthma. *Acta Allergologica* 1972; **27**: 397–400.
7 Schatz M, Patterson R, Zeitz S, O'Rourke J, Melam H. Corticosteroid therapy for the pregnant asthmatic patient. *JAMA* 1975; **233**: 804–7.
8 Fitzsimons R, Greenberger PA, Patterson R. Outcome of pregnancy in women requiring corticosteroids for severe asthma. *J Allergy Clin Immunol* 1986; **78**: 349–53.
9 Doucette JT, Bracken MB. Possible role of asthma in the risk of preterm labor and delivery. *Epidemiology* 1993; **4**: 143–50.

10 Perlow JH, Montgomery D, Morgan MA, Towers CV, Porto M. Severity of asthma and perinatal outcome. *Am J Obstet Gynecol* 1992; **167**: 963–7.
11 Greenberger PA, Patterson R. The outcome of pregnancy complicated by severe asthma. *Allergy Proc* 1988; **9**: 539–43.
12 Schatz M, Zeiger RS, Hoffman CP. Intrauterine growth is related to gestational pulmonary function in pregnant asthmatic women. Kaiser-Permanente asthma and pregnancy study group. *Chest* 1990; **98**: 389–92.
13 Lehrer S, Stone J, Lapinski R, Lockwood CJ, Schachter BS, Berkowitz R, *et al*. Association between pregnancy-induced hypertension and asthma. *Am J Obstet Gynecol* 1993; **168**: 1463–6.
14 Steenius-Aarniala B, Piirila P, Teramo K. Asthma and pregnancy: a prospective study of 198 pregnancies. *Thorax* 1988; **43**: 12–8.
15 Schatz M, Zeiger RS, Hoffman CP, Saunders BS, Harden KM, Forsythe AB. Increased transient tachypnoea of the newborn in infants of asthmatic mothers. *Am J Dis Child* 1991; **145**: 156–8.
16 Patterson CA, Graves WL, Bugg G, Sasso SC, Brann AW Jr. Antenatal and intrapartum factors associated with the occurrence of seizures in term infant. *Obstet Gynecol* 1989; **74**: 361–5.
17 Moore-Gillon JC. Asthma in pregnancy. *Contemp Rev Obstet Gynaecol* 1993; **5**: 25–9.
18 British Thoracic Society. Guidelines for the management of asthma: a summary. *BMJ* 1993; **306**: 776–82.
19 Beasley R, Cushley M, Holgate ST. A self-management plan in the treatment of adult asthma. *Thorax* 1989; **44**: 200–4.
20 Charlton I, Charlton G, Broomfield J, Mullee MA. Evaluation of peak flow and symptom only self management plans for control of asthma in general practice. *BMJ* 1990; **301**: 1355–9.
21 Fainstat T. Cortisone-induced congenital cleft palate in rabbits. *Endocrinology* 1954; **55**: 502.
22 Snyder RD, Snyder D. Corticosteroids for asthma during pregnancy. *Ann Allergy* 1978; **41**: 340–1.
23 Arad I, Landau H. Adrenocortical reserve of neonates born of long-term, steroid-treated mothers. *Eur J Pediatr* 1984; **142**: 279–80.
24 Harris DM. Some properties of beclomethasone dipropionate and related steroids in man. *Postgrad Med J* 1975; **51**: 20–5.
25 Marion-Brown H, Storey G. Beclomethasone dipropionate aerosol in long-term treatment of perennial and seasonal asthma in children and adults. A report of five and a half years experience in 600 asthmatic patients. *Br J Clin Pharmacol* 1977; **4**: 529–67S.
26 Greenberger P, Patterson R. Beclomethasone dipropionate for severe asthma during pregnancy. *Ann Intern Med* 1983; **98**: 478–80.
27 Morgan DJ. Clinical pharmacokinetics of beta-agonists. *Clin Pharmacokinet* 1990; **18**: 270–94.
28 Schatz M, Zeiger RS, Harden KM, *et al*. The safety of inhaled β agonist bronchodilators during pregnancy. *J Allergy Clin Immunol* 1988; **82**: 686–95.
29 Fitzpatrick MF, Mackay T, Driver H, Douglas NJ. Salmeterol in nocturnal asthma: a double blind, placebo controlled trial of a long acting inhaled β_2 agonist. *BMJ* 1990; **301**: 1365–8.
30 Wilson J. Utilisation du cromoglycate de sodium au cours de la grossesse. *Acta Ther* 1982; **8**: 45–51.
31 *British National Formulary*. No 26. London: British Medical Association, Royal Pharmaceutical Society of Great Britain, 1993: 104.
32 Labovitz E, Spector S. Parental theophylline transfer in pregnant asthmatics. *JAMA* 1982; **247**: 786–8.
33 Greenberger P, Patterson R. Safety of therapy for allergic symptoms during pregnancy. *Ann Intern Med* 1978; **89**: 234–7.
34 Heinonen DP, Stone D, Shapiro S. *Birth defects and drugs in pregnancy*. Littleton, MA: Publishing Sciences Group, 1977.
35 Park JM, Schmer V, Myers TL. Cardiovascular anomalies associated with prenatal exposure to theophylline. *South Med J* 1990; **83**: 1487–8.
36 Carter BL, Driscoll CF, Smith GD. Theophylline clearance during pregnancy. *Obstet Gynaecol* 1986; **88**: 146–9.
37 Frederikson MC, Ruo TI, Chow MJ, *et al*. Theophylline pharmacokinetics in pregnancy. *Clin Pharmacol Ther* 1986; **40**: 321–8.

38 Gardner MJ, Schatz M, Cousins L *et al. Longitudinal effects of pregnancy on the pharmacokinetics of theophylline. Eur J Clin Pharmacol* 1987; **31**: 289–95.

39 CLASP (Collaborative low-dose aspirin study in pregnancy) Collaborative Group. CLASP: a randomised trial of low-dose aspirin for the prevention and treatment of pre-eclampsia among 9364 pregnant women. *Lancet* 1994; **343**: 616–29.

40 Broussard RC, Payne DK, George RB. Treatment with acyclovir of varicella pneumonia during pregnancy. *Chest* 1991; **99**: 1045–7.

41 Parayani SG, Arvin AM. Intrauterine infection with varicella-zoster virus after maternal varicella. *N Engl J Med* 1986; **314**: 1542–6.

42 Rice P, Simmons K, Carr R, Banatvala J. Near fatal chickenpox during prednisolone treatment. *BMJ* 1994; **309**: 1069–70.

43 Department of Health, Welsh Office, Scottish Home and Health department and Department of Health and Social Services, Northern Ireland. *Confidential enquiries into maternal deaths in the United Kingdom 1988–90*. London: HMSO, 1994.

44 Fishburne JI Jr, Brenner WE, Braaksma JT, Hendricks CH. Bronchospasm complicating intravenous prostaglandin $F_{2\alpha}$ for therapeutic abortion. *Obstet Gynecol* 1972; **39**: 892–6.

45 Hyman AL, Spannhake EW, Kadowitz QJ. Prostaglandins and the lung: state of the art. *Am Rev Respir Dis* 1978; **117**: 111–36.

46 Gruskay FL. Comparison of breast, cow, and soy feedings in the prevention of onset of allergic disease: a 15-year prospective study. *Clin Pediatr Phil* 1982; **21**: 486–91.

47 Saarinen UM, Kajosaari M, Backman A, Simmes MA. Prolonged breast feeding as prophylaxis for atopic disease. *Lancet* 1979; ii: 163–6.

48 McKenzie SA, Selley JA, Agnew JE. Secretion of prednisolone into breast milk. *Arch Dis Child* 1975; **50**: 894–6.

49 Katz FH, Duncan BR. Entry of prednisolone into human milk. *N Engl J Med* 1975; **293**: 1154.

50 Yurchek AM, Jusko WJ. Theophylline secretion into breast milk. *Pediatrics* 1976; **57**: 518.

6 Treatment of rheumatic diseases

MARGARET A BYRON

Musculoskeletal disorders are very common, accounting for nearly a fifth of all consultations in general practice.[1] Some conditions, such as low back pain and carpal tunnel syndrome, may require treatment during pregnancy, and other specific rheumatological conditions, such as systemic lupus erythematosus and rheumatoid arthritis, have their peak incidence in women of childbearing age.

An adequate explanation of the risks of any proposed treatment, with appropriate advice on contraception, is essential when treating women of childbearing age. In women with established rheumatic diseases it is important to appreciate that, without the use of drugs which suppress the disease, pregnancy may not occur or may not be carried to term. Adequate control of the disease may also enable a woman to feel capable of bearing and raising children. There is a good chance of remission of rheumatoid arthritis during pregnancy, though for systemic lupus erythematosus aggressive treatment may continue to be necessary.[2] The use of drugs that pose the least threat to the fetus will minimise anxiety, should pregnancy occur.

Box 6.1 lists the drugs prescribed for rheumatic conditions; two recent reviews examined the effects of these drugs in pregnancy and lactation.[3,4] Analgesics and non-steroidal anti-inflammatory drugs are most commonly prescribed and also account for a large proportion of self prescription (over the counter) drugs. In a recent study in Cape Town, 29% of pregnant women self prescribed and 60% did not know that certain medicines are

---

Box 6.1   Drugs used for rheumatological conditions

Analgesics Non-steroidal anti-inflammatory drugs	Soft tissue lesions Inflammatory arthritis Osteoarthritis Non-specific back pain
Disease modifying antirheumatic drugs	
Sulphasalazine	Rheumatoid arthritis Ankylosing spondylitis
Antimalarials	Systemic lupus erythematosus Rheumatoid arthritis
Gold salts Penicillamine	Rheumatoid arthritis Psoriatic arthritis

Immunosuppressive drugs:
  Cytotoxic agents
    Methotrexate   Severe unremitting rheumatoid arthritis
    Azathioprine   Systemic lupus erythematosus
    Cyclophosphamide   Other connective tissue diseases
  Corticosteroids   Systemic lupus erythematosus
                       Other connective tissue diseases
                       Rheumatoid arthritis
  Cyclosporin   Severe unremitting rheumatoid arhtritis
                       Psoriatic arthritis

---

unsafe in pregnancy.[5] It cannot therefore be assumed that women are always aware of the risks.

Analgesics

Analgesics are commonly prescribed and bought over the counter during pregnancy, especially paracetamol. This crosses the placenta easily but does not seem to be associated with fetal malformations.[3,4,6] Codeine also seems safe in pregnancy, though neonatal drug withdrawal syndrome has been described with codeine and dextropropoxyphene.[4] Even with established inflammatory arthritis, well motivated women with moderate symptoms may be managed with simple analgesics, paracetamol being the drug of choice.

Breast feeding – Paracetamol is excreted in small amounts in breast milk but is a safe analgesic to use during lactation.[7] Although codeine is lipid soluble and might concentrate in breast milk, it is considered safe in breast feeding.

Non-steroidal anti-inflammatory drugs

These are first line agents in treating inflammatory poly-arthritis. For soft tissue and degenerative conditions, anti-inflammatory drugs should be prescribed only for the short term. Analgesics should be used if possible.

Teratogenicity – Animal studies have linked a variety of skeletal and craniovertebral abnormalities with ingestion of large doses of salicylates during pregnancy. In humans several retrospective surveys have shown that significantly more mothers of malformed infants took salicylates regularly during pregnancy than mothers of normal infants. These findings have not been corroborated in prospective studies.[8–11] The largest study, the Perinatal Colla-borative Project in the United States, found that malformation rates were similar in the children of 35 418 women not exposed to aspirin, 9736 with intermediate exposure, and 5128 heavily exposed during the first four months of pregnancy.[11] Overall, therefore, the evidence suggests that salicylates used in recommended doses are unlikely to produce fetal malformation. Diflunisal, a salicylic acid derivative, has been shown to be teratogenic in animals at very high doses, but no such abnormalities have been reported in humans.[12]

Other non-steroidal anti-inflammatory drugs have not been as well studied as aspirin. Teratogenicity has been reported in animals given indomethacin, diclofenac, and azapropazone, though the doses received far exceed those given to humans. The only reports of fetal malformation in humans are two anecdotal case reports implicating indomethacin.[3]

There is little information on the newer anti-inflammatories, such as etodolac or nabumetone, but no evidence of teratogenicity has been found with commonly prescribed propionic acid derivatives such as ibuprofen, ketoprofen, flurbiprofen, fenopro-fen, and naproxen. Phenylbutazone is best avoided in pregnancy as it has been associated with chromosomal abnormalities in adults.[3,4]

Fetal growth retardation – A survey from Sydney showed that long term ingestion of aspirin was associated with an increased incidence of stillbirth and reduced birth weight compared with that of controls.[10] Most of the aspirin preparations ingested, however, were compounds containing substances such as phenacetin and caffeine and were taken in large doses. Data from the United States showed no significant effect of aspirin ingestion on birth weight and perinatal mortality.[8,11,12] There is no convincing evidence that indomethacin or other non-steroidal anti-inflammatory agents affect fetal growth.

Effects mediated through inhibition of prostaglandin synthesis – All non-steroidal anti-inflammatory drugs reduce inflammation by inhibiting prostaglandin synthesis to varying degrees. As prostaglandins play a major role in fetal development, their inhibition has various effects on the mother, fetus and neonate (box 6.2).

A retrospective study of women with musculoskeletal disorders showed that those who took more than 3·25 g of aspirin a day during the last six months of pregnancy had a significantly longer gestation, longer labour, and greater blood loss at delivery than women who had not taken aspirin.[13,14] Turner and Collins also found an increased incidence of anaemia, antepartum haemorrhage, and pre-eclampsia in women who took aspirin for long periods.[10] Haemostatic abnormalities and a higher incidence of

---

Box 6.2   Conditions associated with use of inhibitors of prostaglandin synthesis in pregnancy

Effects on mother:
- Prolongation of pregnancy
- Prolongation of labour
- Increased blood loss both before and after birth
- Anaemia
- Pre-eclampsia

Effects on fetus and neonate:
- Haemostatic abnormalities
- Increased incidence of intracranial haemorrhage
- Premature closure of ductus arteriosus
- Persistent pulmonary hypertension

---

intracranial haemorrhage have been found in neonates whose mothers ingested aspirin within a few days before delivery.[15,16]

In the fetus, prostaglandin E causes relaxation of systemic and pulmonary vessels as well as the ductus arteriosus, and 90% of blood ejected by the right ventricle passes through the ductus arteriosus to the descending aorta.[17] In a variety of animals, administration of single doses of an anti-inflammatory agent results in reversible constriction of the ductus arteriosus and a substantial increase in pulmonary artery pressure in the fetus. Long term exposure to anti-inflammatory agents in animals and humans is associated with increased amounts of pulmonary artery smooth muscle, which results in persistent pulmonary hypertension in the newborn infant, with or without premature closure of the ductus arteriosus.[18]

Indomethacin has been used for the treatment of preterm labour. Babies born preterm after exposure to indomethacin given for this indication have a high neonatal morbidity, with necrotising enterocolitis, intracranial haemorrhage, and patent ductus arteriosus.[19] It is likely that the dose and duration of administration of the drug, the gestational age of the fetus at the time of exposure, and the time between the last dose of the drug and the birth of the infant are important factors. Infants born to mothers receiving long term anti-inflammatory treatment are probably most at risk. The most potent inhibitors of prostaglandin synthesis — salicylates and indomethacin, for example — should be avoided throughout pregnancy and certainly during the last trimester. To minimise the effects on the fetus, drugs with a short elimination half life and inactive metabolites — such as ibuprofen, flurbiprofen, and ketoprofen — should be used at the maximum tolerated dosage interval.

The synthetic prostaglandin analogue misoprostol is licensed for use as a mucosal protective agent in combination with anti-inflammatory drugs. It can also be coprescribed with either naproxen (a combined pack) or diclofenac (a combined tablet). As misoprostol increases uterine tone, it should be avoided in women of childbearing age unless adequate contraception is being used.

Breast feeding – Because non-steroidal anti-inflammatory drugs are weak acids they do not achieve high concentrations in milk. All manufacturers state in their drug information that these drugs should not be used in lactating women. This caution is based on lack of specific information rather than known adverse reactions, and the benefit associated with breast feeding may outweigh the risks of a carefully chosen drug. The appropriate drugs should have a short elimination half life and metabolites which are inert or rapidly eliminated or both. Hydroxy or methyl metabolites are relatively stable in the infant's stomach, whereas glucuronide derivatives may be cleaved, releasing active metabolites.[3] Boxes 6.3 and 6.4 show the suitability of various drugs. Reported side effects are uncommon, but plasma salicylate concentrations of 1·74 mmol/l (24 mg/dl) were found in a breast fed child with metabolic acidosis whose mother was taking 2·4 g aspirin a day, and a grand mal fit occurred in a child whose mother was taking indomethacin.[3]

Disease modifying drugs

The drugs discussed in this section are second line agents for

---

Box 6.3 Suitable drugs for use during lactation

Analgesics
Paracetamol   } see text
Codeine

Non-steroidal anti-inflammatory drugs:

Ibuprofen   Small quantities in milk
Flurbiprofen   Short elimination half life
Diclofenac   Inert metabolites
Mefenamic acid

Naproxen   Small quantities in milk
    Little ingestion by infant

Fenoprofen   Very small quantities in milk
Ketoprofen   Short elimination half life
    Glucuronide metabolites not important
    here

Piroxocam   Only 1–3% of maternal plasma
    consentrationa in breast milk despite
    long half life

Disease modifying drugs:
Sulphasalazine   See text

Immunosuppressive drugs:
Corticosteroids   See text

Box 6.4   Unsuitable drugs during lactation

Non-steroidal anti-inflammatory drugs:

Salicylates	Glucuronide metabolites Risk of Reye's syndrome
Diflunisal Tolmetin Azapropazone }	Long half life
Febufen Sulindac }	Active metabolites
Indomethacin	Variable half life; enterohepatic circulation of metabolites

Disease modifying drugs:

Antimalarials	Risk of retinal damage
Gold salts d-Penicillamine }	Potential renal and bone marrow toxicity

Immunosuppressive drugs:

Cytotoxic agents Cyclosporin }	See text

---

the treatment of inflammatory polyarthritis, and there is a trend for starting them earlier in the course of rheumatoid arthritis to prevent joint destruction and disability. The immunosuppressive drugs are most often used for connective tissue diseases and vasculitis.

Sulphasalazine

Sulphasalazine is well established as a second line treatment for rheumatoid arthritis. The drug reversibly reduces male sperm count but does not seem to affect female fertility. Experience of its use in the treatment of inflammatory bowel disease has shown it to be safe throughout pregnancy and lactation.[3,20,21] There is a theoretical risk of neonatal haemolysis and two case reports describe diarrhoea developing in breast fed infants.[22,23] As sulphasalazine impairs absorption of folate, supplementation is recommended in pregnancy.

Antimalarial drugs

Chloroquine salts cross the placenta and rapidly accumulate in mouse fetal tissues such as the eye.[24] Teratogenic effects are probably related to dose. Prophylactic treatment of malaria during pregnancy seems safe,[25] but exposure during the first trimester to the doses of chloroquine required to treat rheumatic diseases has been associated with sensorineural hearing loss in an infant.[26] Two recent studies reviewed a total of 41 pregnancies in 32 women treated with chloroquine salts.[27,28] Twenty pregnancies resulted in normal babies, and the 21 fetal losses seemed to be related to disease activity rather than to treatment. In Levy's review of 215 pregnancies in women exposed to chloroquine, seven fetuses (3·3%) had congenital abnormalities.

The theoretical risk from antimalarials suggests that women should be advised to avoid pregnancy while taking chloroquine salts, but the clinical evidence shows no reason to withdraw chloroquine during pregnancy in rheumatoid arthritis or systemic lupus erythematosus if the disease process is controlled. Women can be reassured that pregnancy outcome is likely to be normal.

Breast feeding – Both chloroquine and hydroxychloroquine have been found in small quantities in human milk, and the authors of one study predicted that an infant would be exposed to about 2% of the maternal dose per day.[29] Despite the lack of reported adverse effects in breast fed infants of women receiving malaria prophylaxis, caution is advised when the drugs are used in the higher doses required for treating chronic rheumatic conditions. As potential retinal damage would be difficult to monitor in children of this age, chloroquine salts are not recommended for use in lactating women.

Gold salts

Both gold thiomalate and auranofin, an oral gold preparation, have proved teratogenic in animals.[3] Gold has been found in the liver and kidneys of an aborted human fetus, and there are reports of possible teratogenic effects.[30,31] Other studies report the safe use of gold in pregnancy, and therapeutic gold concentrations have been detected in cord blood without evidence of congenital defects.[32] Similarly, no adverse reactions occurred in 13 mothers or their infants treated with auranofin throughout pregnancy.[33] There is therefore no hard evidence to suggest withdrawing treatment with gold during pregnancy if it is controlling disease. It is sensible to reduce the dose and frequency of administration.

Breast feeding – Trace amounts of gold salts have been detected in the milk of lactating women,[34] and more recently gold has been detected in the serum of suckling infants.[35] Calculations of the weight adjusted dose indicated that the dose to the infant exceeded that received by the mother. The theoretical possibility of gold toxicity precludes its use during breast feeding.

d-Penicillamine

The chelating agent d-penicillamine is used to treat Wilson's disease, cystinuria, and rheumatoid arthritis. It crosses the placenta and is potentially teratogenic. Its use in pregnancy has been associated with the development of a generalised connective tissue defect similar to Ehlers-Danlos syndrome,[36–39] which in some cases was found to be reversible. Many women with Wilson's disease have given birth to normal infants despite large doses of d-penicillamine throughout pregnancy,[40,41] and it has been proposed that in this disease the fetus is protected from the effects of pencillamine by the excessive maternal pool of copper. In two other surveys, however, a ventricular septal defect was the only abnormality reported in women with rheumatoid arthritis and cystinuria.[42,43] About 90 cases of taking penicillamine in pregnancy have been reported,[4] and the evidence suggests continuing penicillamine in Wilson's disease where the benefits of treatment cut the risks to the fetus, but discontinuing it where safer alternative drugs are available.

Breast feeding – No data are available on excretion of d-penicillamine in breast milk. The potential toxicity makes its use hazardous.

Immunosuppressive drugs

Cytotoxic agents

The antimetabolite methotrexate is being used increasingly to control rheumatoid and psoriatic arthritis; the alkylating agents cyclophosphamide and chlorambucil are used rarely. All three are considered teratogenic and mutagenic, and even if cytotoxic agents are used after the first trimester the fetus is susceptible to bone marrow depression, infection, and haemorrhage.[44] Experience with low dose methotrexate for rheumatoid arthritis is accumulating, but little has been reported about its use in pregnancy. A small uncontrolled study of 10 pregnancies in eight women who took methotrexate early in pregnancy failed to show teratogenicity but suggested that the risk of spontaneous abortion may be increased.[45] No long term effects were seen in the five offspring (mean age at follow up 11·5 years).

Increasing numbers of normal pregnancy outcomes have been described in women taking azathioprine (a cytotoxic immunosuppressant),[46,47] though some infants have had lymphopenia, growth retardation, and an increase in chromosomal breakages. Results of a larger, longer term, follow up study are encouraging, though mean follow up of the children was only six years (range 5–13 years).[48] No increase in fetal abnormalities or abortion rate has been recorded in patients who remain fertile after cytotoxic chemotherapy. Ideally, cytotoxic agents should be discontinued some time before conception is contemplated, but azathioprine may need to be continued during pregnancy to prevent a flare of the underlying disease.

Breast feeding – Cyclophosphamide and methotrexate are found in human breast milk and the potential risk to the infant precludes their use.[4] There are no data on azathioprine.

Cyclosporin

Cyclosporin is a fungal metabolite and a potent immunosuppressant. The experience of cyclosporin use during pregnancy in women who had received kidney transplants has established its safety, and case reports in other conditions (lupus nephritis, for example) are supportive.[49] It is excreted in breast milk, and the manufacturers recommend avoiding its use during lactation.

Corticosteroids

These drugs are discussed more fully in the chapter on asthma. Several studies have confirmed the low risk to the fetus and mother with a rheumatic disorder of taking corticosteroids in pregnancy.[50–52] Additional doses of steroid are needed to cover delivery, but fetal adrenal insufficiency has not been described.

Breast feeding – In the doses most commonly used for treating rheumatic disorders (15 mg of prednisolone or less a day) there is little chance of the infant receiving significant amounts of prednisolone in breast milk.[53]

Summary

The outlook for successful pregnancy in women with rheumatic diseases has improved in the past 10 years. With appropriate information and advice before conception, the risks to mother, fetus, and neonate can be minimised.

Key points

- In rheumatic diseases drugs might be required to enable a woman to become pregnant

- Analgesics and anti-inflammatory agents are often self prescribed

- Paracetamol is safe in pregnancy and lactation

- Indomethacin has major adverse effects in both preterm and term babies

- Non-steroidal anti-inflammatory drugs used in pregnancy and lactation should be those with a short half life and inactive metabolites – ibuprofen, for example

- Sulphasalazine is safe in pregnancy and lactation

- Gold and penicillamine are relatively safe in pregnancy but their doses should be reduced

- Cytotoxic drugs should be discontinued before pregnancy

- Azathioprine, cyclosporin, and steroids are relatively safe in pregnancy and might be needed to control the underlying disease

- Breast feeding should be avoided if taking antimalarial drugs, gold, penicillamine, cytotoxic drugs, or cyclosporin

- Prednisolone is safe in pregnancy and lactation

1 Office of Population Censuses and Surveys. *Morbidity statistics from general practice: third national survey.* London: HMSO, 1986.
2 Dudley DJ, Branch DW. Pregnancy in the patient with rheumatic disease: the obstetrician's perspective. In: Parke AL, ed. *Clinical rheumatology.* London: Baillière Tindall, 1990; 4: 141–56.
3 Brooks PM, Needs CJ. Antirheumatic drugs in pregnancy and lactation. In: Parke AL, ed. *Clinical Rheumatology.* London: Baillière Tindall, 1990; 4: 157–71.
4 Keen WF, Buchanan WW. Pregnancy and rheumatoid disease. In: Parke AL, ed. *Clinical Rheumatology.* London: Baillière Tindall, 1990; 4: 125–40.
5 Aviv RI, Chubb K, Lindow SW. The prevalence of maternal medication ingestion in the antenatal period. *S Afr Med J* 1993; 83: 657–60.
6 Aselton P, Jick H, Milunsky A, Hunter JR, Stergachis A. First trimester drug use and congenital disorders. *Obstet Gynaecol* 1985; 65: 451–5.
7 Bitzen PO, Gustaffson B, Jostell KG, *et al.* Excretion of paracetamol in human breast milk. *Eur J Clin Pharmacol* 1981; 20: 123–5.

8 Collins E. Maternal and fetal effects of acetaminophen and salicylates in pregnancy. *Obstet Gynaecol* 1981; **58 (suppl 5)**: 57–62.

9 Buckfield P. Major congenital faults in newborn infants: a pilot study in New Zealand. *NZ Med J* 1973; **78**: 195–204.

10 Turner G, Collins E. Fetal effects of regular salicylate ingestion in pregnancy. *Lancet* 1975; ii: 338–40.

11 Slone D, Heinonen OP, Kaufman DW, Siskind V, Monson RR, Shapiro S. Aspirin and congenital malformations. *Lancet* 1976; i: 1373–5.

12 Shapiro S, Monson R, Kaufman DW, Siskind V, Heinonen OP, Slone D. Perinatal mortality and birth weight in relation to aspirin taken during pregnancy. *Lancet* 1976; i: 1375–6.

13 Lewis RB, Shulman JD. Influence of acetylsalicylic acid, an inhibitor of prostaglandin synthesis, on the duration of human gestation and labour. *Lancet* 1973; ii: 1159–61.

14 Lee P. Anti-inflammatory therapy during pregnancy and lactation. *Clin Invest Med* 1985; **8**: 328–33.

15 Rumack CM, Guggenheim MA, Rumack BH, Peterson RG, Johnson ML, Braithwaite WR. Neonatal intracranial haemorrhage and maternal use of aspirin. *Obstet Gynaecol* 1981; **58 (suppl 5)**: 52–6.

16 Stuart MJ, Gross SJ, Elrad H, Graeber JE. Effects of acetylsalicylic-acid ingestion on maternal and neonatal hemostasis. *N Engl J Med* 1982; **307**: 909–12.

17 Rudolph AM. The effects of non-steroidal anti-inflammatory compounds on fetal circulation and pulmonary function. *Obstet Gynaecol* 1981; **58** (suppl 5): 63–7.

18 Levin DL, Mills LJ, Weinberg AG. Haemodynamic pulmonary vasculature and myocardial abnormalities secondary to pharmacologic constriction of fetus ductus arteriosus: a possible mechanism for persistent pulmonary hypertension and transient tricuspid insufficiency in the new born infant. *Circulation* 1979; **60**: 360–4.

19 Norton ME, Merrill J, Cooper BAB, Kuller JA, Clyman RI. Neonatal complications after the administration of indomethacin for preterm labor. *N Engl J Med* 1993; **329**: 1602–7.

20 Vender RJ, Spiro HW. Inflammatory bowel disease and pregnancy. *J Clin Gastroenterol* 1982; **4**: 231–49.

21 Newman NM, Correy JF. Possible teratogenicity of sulphasalazine. *Med J Austr* 1983; ii: 528–9.

22 Branski D, Kerem E, Gross-Kieselstein E, Hurvitz H, Litt R, Abrahamov A. Bloody diarrhoea – a possible complication of sulfasalazine transferred through human breast milk. *J Pediat Gastroenterol Nutr* 1986; **5**: 316–7.

23 Nelis GF. Diarrhoea due to 5-aminosalicylic acid in breast milk. *Lancet* 1989; i: 383.

24 Ullberg S. Lindquist N, Sjostrand S. Accumulation of chorio-retinotoxic drugs in the foetal eye. *Nature* 1970; **227**: 1257–8.

25 Lewis R, Laursen NH, Birnbaum S. Malaria associated with pregnancy. *Obstet Gynaecol* 1973; **42**: 696–700.

26 Hart CW, Naunton RF. The ototoxicity of chloroquine phosphate. *Arch Otolaryngol* 1964; **80**: 407–12.

27 Parke AL. Anti-malarial drugs. Systemic lupus erythematosus and pregnancy. *J Rheumatol* 1988; **15**: 607–10.

28 Levy M, Buskila D, Gladman DD, Urowitz MB, Koren G. Pregnancy outcome following first trimester exposure to chloroquine. *Am J Perinatol* 1991; **8**: 174–8.

29 Nation RL, Hacket LP, Dusci LJ, *et al.* Excretion of hydroxychloroquine in human milk. *Br J Clin Pharmacol* 1984; **17**: 368–9.

30 Rocker I, Henderson WJ. Transfer of gold from mother to fetus. *Lancet* 1976; ii: 1246.

31 Rogers JG, Anderson RMcD, Chow CW. Possible teratogenic effects of gold. *Aust Paediatr J* 1980; **16**: 195–8.

32 Cohen DL, Orzd J, Taylor A. Infants of mothers receiving gold therapy. *Arthritis Rheum* 1981; **24**: 104–5.

33 Ostensen M, Husby G. Antirheumatic drug treatment during pregnancy and lactation. *Scand J Rheum* 1985; **14**: 1–7.

34 Ostensen M, Skavdal K, Myklebust G, *et al.* Excretion of gold in human breast milk. *Eur J Clin Pharmacol* 1986; **31**: 261.

35 Bennett PN, Humphries SJ, Osborne JP, Clarke AK, Taylor A. Use of sodium aurothiomalate during lactation. *Br J Clin Pharmacol* 1990; **29**: 777–9.

36 Mjolnerod OK, Dommerud SA, Rasmussen K, Gjeruldsen ST. Congenital connective tissue defect probably due to d-pencillamine treatment in pregnancy. *Lancet* 1971; i: 673–5.

37 Solomon L, Abrahams G, Dinner M, Berman L. Neonatal abnormalities associated with d-penicillamine treatment during pregnancy. *N Engl J Med* 1977; **296**: 54–5.

38 Linares A, Zarranz JJ, Rodriguez-Alarcon J, Diaz-Perez JL. Reversible cutis laxa due to maternal d-penicillamine therapy. *Lancet* 1979; ii: 43.
39 Rosa FW. Teratogen update: penicillamine. *Teratology* 1986; **33**: 127–31.
40 Scheinberg IH, Sternlieb I. Pregnancy in penicillamine treated patients with Wilson's disease. *N Engl J Med* 1975; **293**: 1300–2.
41 Walshe JM. Pregnancy in Wilson's disease. *Q J Med* 1977; **46**: 73–83.
42 Lyle WH. Penicillamine in pregnancy. *Lancet* 1978; i: 606–7.
43 Gregory MC, Mansell MA. Pregnancy and cystinuria. *Lancet* 1983; ii:1158–60.
44 Barber HRK. Fetal and neonatal effects of cytotoxic agents. *Obstet Gynaecol* 1981; **58** (suppl 5): 41–7.
45 Kozlowski RD, Steinbrunner JV, MacKenzie AM, *et al.* Outcome of first trimester exposure to low-dose methotrexate in eight patients with rheumatic disease. *Am J Med* 1990; **88**: 589–92.
46 Nolan GH, Sweet RL, Laros RK. Renal cadaver transplantation followed by successful pregnancies. *Obstet Gynecol* 1974; **4**: 732–9.
47 Hayslett JP, Lynn RI. Effect of pregnancy in patients with lupus nephropathy. *Kidney International* 1980; **18**: 207–20.
48 Ramsey-Goldman R, Mientus JM, Kutzer JE, Mulvihill JJ, Medsger TA. Pregnancy outcome in women with systemic lupus erythematosus treated with immunosuppressive drugs. *J Rheumatol* 1993; **20**: 1152–7.
49 Hussein MM, Mooij JM, Roujouleh H. Cyclosporine in the treatment of lupus nephritis including two patients treated during pregnancy. *Clin Nephrol* 1993; **40**: 160–3.
50 Popert AJ. Pregnancy and adrenocortical hormones: some aspects of their interactions in rheumatic diseases. *BMJ* 1962; i: 967–72.
51 Yackel DB, Kempers RD, McConahey WM. Adrenocorticosteroid therapy in pregnancy. *Am J Obstet Gynecol* 1966; **96**: 985–9.
52 Grigor RR, Shervington PC, Hughes GRV, *et al.* Outcome of pregnancy in systemic lupus erythematosus. *Proc R Soc Med* 1977; **70**: 99–100.
53 McKenzie SA, Selley JA, Agnew JE. Secretion of prednisolone into breast milk. *Arch Dis Child* 1975; **50**: 894–6.

7 Psychotropic drugs

JB LOUDON

Introduction

At some time during their pregnancy about 20% of a random sample of women attending antenatal clinics will experience significant psychological distress, mainly anxiety.[1] Risk factors include previous psychologial illness, previous termination of pregnancy, adverse social backgrounds, and single parenthood.[2]

Few women are referred to a psychiatrist during pregnancy. This reflects a referral bias rather than any epidemiological truth. In a comparison with non-pregnant controls, pregnant women were shown to have a higher rate of morbidity.[3] During the puerperium, 0.2% of mothers will develop psychotic illness, at least 10% will develop a depressive illness, and a further 16% will have a self limiting depressive reaction (lasting up to a month). Often these depressive illnesses and reactions are not reported to the patient's general practitioner, but they are corrosive to personal wellbeing, to marital happiness, and to enjoyment of mothering. They merit attention and appropriate treatment. In one sample of pregnant women with severe depressive disorders, 50% remained unwell for a year and few had received sustained treatment.[2]

The distress of pregnancy, being related to adverse events or social circumstances, is not easily treated with drugs. The disorders of the puerperium seem to be caused by a biological disturbance but occur more often in primigravids, in unmarried women, in those who have had a caesarean section, and after a perinatal death. In these cases drug treatment is indicated.[4]

This article discusses psychotropic drugs but it should be

remembered that other forms of treatment are important. These include support from staff or self help groups, psychological treatments such as relaxation exercises or cognitive therapy, and mobilisation of community resources.

Psychotropic drugs

Psychotropic drugs differ from other medications in several respects. Their onset of action tends to be delayed, two to three weeks in the case of antidepressants and for up to one month for antipsychotic drugs. Similarly, a rebound of illness may not follow drug withdrawal for quite some time owing to the vagaries of tissue storage; it may be quite difficult for a patient to appreciate the connection. Many of the older psychotropic drugs have a range of side effects, but there is more experience of their use than of the newer, "cleaner" psychotropic agents, which cannot be recommended yet for use in pregnancy because their toxicity is not known.

For the older antidepressant and antipsychotic drugs, the dose required for successful treatment may vary 10-fold, requiring careful titration to the patient's illness. Benzodiazepines can produce physical dependence if taken longer than one month. This risk has been well publicised in the past decade, and the opprobrium has tended to generalise to all psychotropics, quite unjustifiably, so that it has become more difficult to persuade patients to start and stay on antidepressant treatment. Relatives and neighbours may consider themselves expert on psychotropic drugs and offer advice on dosage and compliance. Worse, they may act as additional sources of supply, unknown to the doctor.

Psychotropic drugs used in pregnancy and during the peurperium

- the hypnotic and anxiolytic drugs
- neuroleptic drugs
- antidepressants
- lithium carbonate
- anticonvulsants used in mood regulation

Safety of psychotropic drugs used in pregnancy and during the puerperium

Hypnotics and anxiolytics: benzodiazepines

Only benzodiazepine drugs should be used; barbiturates and the older anxiolytics drugs such as meprobamate are obsolete. Reports from Scandinavia in the early 1970s suggested that children of mothers who used benzodiazepines were more likely to have defects of the palate, but other studies at the time failed to confirm the finding. A careful study that compared 611 infants with such deformities and 2498 controls found no evidence of an excess of diazepam use by their mothers.[5] Some reassurance about this risk can therefore be given to an anxious woman who has been taking diazepam in early pregnancy. Use of benzodiazepines in the first three months of pregnancy is associated with the occurrence of pyloric stenosis, cardiac defects, and inguinal hernias, concomitant smoking increases the risk nearly fourfold.[6] One study, of eight infants who had been exposed to benzodiazepines throughout gestation, showed a high incidence of craniofacial defects, growth retardation, and learning disability.[7]

Abrupt withdrawal of diazepam during pregnancy is not justified in the light of the well attested likelihood (40% to 50%) of a withdrawl reaction, which may be quite incapacitating and include distorted sensory perceptions. The withdrawal reaction may be worse if the patient is taking benzodiazepines with a short duration of action, metabolised to an inactive compound. She should be switched to chlordiazepoxide, whose active metabolite, desmethyldiazepam, has a long half life; this smooths out symptoms arising from fluctuations in the serum concentration of the drug. Personality factors affect the ease of withdrawal and tolerance of symptoms.[8] Support, education of both patient and partner, relaxation training, and referral to a local support group for tranquilliser dependence will all help.

With a programme of drug reduction, more rapidly to start with and slowly later, written out in advance so the patient knows what is planned, complete withdrawal is possible within 10 days, although circulating drugs may not disappear for another two or three days. Screening urine for metabolites of psychtropic drugs can be used to detect non-compliance with the regimen.

There is no evidence to suggest that benzodiazepines have a harmful effect on the fetus later in pregnancy, but the need for these drugs has to be clear to justify their use, especially on a regular basis. Diazepam appears in fetal blood a few minutes after it has been given to the mother by intravenous or intramuscular injection, and the fetus seems to have a limited capacity to metabolise the drug.[9] Pharmacologically, the fetus acts as a "deep compartment" wherein diazepam is slow to accumulate but also, with its active metabolites, is eliminated slowly. This means that regular ingestion of diazepam by the mother will result in accumulation in the fetus. These factors seem to explain the finding that during labour a single bolus of less than 30 mg of diazepam has no adverse effect on the infant as measured by the Apgar score. A larger single dose or sustained prenatal benzodiazepine can lead to the "floppy infant syndrome," which is characterised by hypotonia, respiratory embarrassment, difficulty in suckling, and hypothermia. There is also good evidence for a withdrawal syndrome in infants whose mothers have taken benzodiazepines regularly during pregnancy.[10]

Diazepam is present in maternal blood un-ionised and is lipophilic; it is therefore readily transferred to breast milk. The newborn infant continues to have an impaired ability to metabolise the drug completely (diazepam has been found in an infant six days after a single dose was given to the mother)[11] and regular use by the mother leads to accumulation in the child. There is little justification for nursing mothers to use diazepam or any of the long acting, older drugs such as chlordiazepoxide or nitrazepam. Though lorazepam has been associated with neonatal hyptonicity, it may not enter breast milk in troublesome amounts. Neonates seem to be able to metabolise oxazepam satisfactorily after the second or third day,[12] which might justify prefering this drug when a nursing mother has to use a benzodiazepine.

Neuroleptic drugs: phenothiazines and thioxanthines

Pregnant women are unlikely to start taking neuroleptic drugs unless they are given as an obsolete and inadvisable treatment for anxiety. Women who have suffered from episodes of a functional psychosis may, however, be receiving long term neuroleptic treatment as prophylaxis and be pregnant owing to neglecting contraceptive measures as a result of the illness or its aftereffects.

At most neuroleptics are highly lipid soluble, the original drug and active metabolites may continue to be excreted for some months after treatment has stopped. This is particularly true of the depot preparations, where the drug is esterified and injected in an oily vehicle to delay adsorption. Stopping such treatment for someone already pregnant will therefore make little immediate difference to the environment of the fetus. Ideally, someone receiving neuroleptics and thinking of becoming pregnant should stop treatment well before conception. This will show the fragility of their wellbeing in the drug free state, as well as minimising exposure of the fetus to the drug. Opinion is shifting towards maintaining patients on lower doses of neuroleptics than hitherto. If conception has taken place a careful reduction in dose could be negotiated with the patient and her general practitioner or psychiatrist, but a subsequent need to treat the relapse resulting from an overenthusiastic pursuit of this goal benefits no one. The puerperium is a time of increased risk of relapse for those who have had a schizophrenic or schizoaffective illness, and continuing drug treatment has some protective effect. A study of schizophrenic mothers showed that neonatal mortality is twice that in normal controls,[13] which makes assessment of the overall danger of neuroleptic drugs more difficult. Several studies have failed to show a teratogenic effect of neuroleptic drugs,[14] especially trifluoperazine,[15] taken in early pregnancy, and no lasting behavioural or developmental effects on the child have been found as a result of exposure to neuroleptics in later pregnancy. Prochlorperazine, which is used more often as antiemetic, was thought to be teratogenic when the fetus is exposed between the sixth and tenth weeks of gestation, but large scale surveillance studies have not confirmed this.[14] Because of its hypotensive actions, chlorpromazine should be avoided immediately before and during delivery.

Neuroleptic drugs enter breast milk in clinically unimportant amounts. Sedation is the commonest reaction in the infant. There are a few reports of a pseudoparkinsonian reaction in neonates born to mothers taking oral or depot neuroleptic drugs.[16]

Tricylic antidepressants

The structure of many neuroleptic drugs is closely related to that of the tricylic antidepressants, and there is much overlap in their pharmacological effects. Not surprisingly, therefore, the information about their use during pregnancy and lactation is similar. The newer non-tricyclic antidepressants are a different matter in that their safety has not yet been proved. Two such drugs (zimelidine and nomofensine) have been withdrawn in the past 15 years because of unexpected toxicity, so, the newer antidepressant drugs are best avoided in pregnancy.

As happens in adults when tricyclics are suddenly withdrawn, a withdrawal reaction has been reported in some neonates born to mothers who received tricyclic antidepressants in the last month of pregnancy.[17] The effects include irritability, apparent abdominal cramps, restlessness, insomnia, and fever.

Little evidence of the use of the monoamine oxidase inhibitors in pregnancy has been published. This reflects the ambiguous position they have held in the antidepressant armoury over the past two decades. One study shows an increased risk of malformations.[18] More recently, there has been something of a reawakening of interest in their use. A new selective monoamine oxidase inhibitor, moclobemide, has been released onto the market. New compounds should not be used in pregnancy, and the older monoamine oxidase inhibitors are best avoided, not because they are known to be toxic but because their interaction with sympathomimetics, β blockers, opiates such as pethidine, and foodstuffs such as cheese causes a potentially fatal hypertension. This makes the anaesthetist's task unenviable. The risk of interaction persists for 10 days after the monoamine oxidase inhibitor is withdrawn, as the enzyme inhibition is irreversible. Another side effect, hypotension, poses a risk to fetal wellbeing.

Both neuroleptic drugs and tricyclic antidepressants enter breast milk in detectable quantities, but ingestion of small amounts of these drugs does not seem to affect the neonate. Indeed, follow up studies over long periods of the children of mothers taking chlorpromazine failed to show any adverse effect on development.[19] There is little published information on the transfer of monoamine oxidase inhibitors to breast milk; tranylcypromine seems to be safe for nursing mothers.[20]

If possible, a patient taking antidepressants long term to prevent a relapse would withdraw gradually from them before becoming pregnant, which has the additional effect of showing her and her partner how robust is her apparent wellbeing. If depressive symptoms return, all concerned will be in a dilemma. For a patient who has suffered a previous major depressive episode, the risk of a recurrence after a subsequent pregnancy is at least 1 in 10. If she enters the pregnancy with symptons or is taking medication to suppress them, the postpartum period is likely to be difficult, but not so difficult as to prohibit pregnancy. Both patient and partner should receive enough information and counselling to allow them to make a choice. There is a good chance that taking an adequate dose of antidepressant will prevent recurrence of depression postpartum. Non-pharmacological treatments such as cognitive behaviour therapy should be borne in mind.

An episode of depressive illness occurring during pregnancy can be treated quite safely with a tricylic antidepressant, preferably at the minimum dose consistent with clinical effectiveness, but the dose required may range from 25 mg to 150 mg of amitriptyline or equivalent. If there is no response at a lower dose, a larger one has to be tried, if antidepressant treatment is worthwhile. The tertiary compounds such as amitriptyline or impipramine often cause side effects such as constipation or postural hypotension. One of the secondary amineses, such as nortriptyline or desipramine, may be preferable. Electroconvulsive therapy may be given during pregnancy for cases that resist treatment without undue hazard to the fetus. The important role of support, counselling, and more specialised psychotherapy should not be forgotten.

Lithium carbonate

Manic-depressive disorder is an illness of young adults, including many women of childbearing age. Many studies have confirmed the teratogenic effect of lithium taken in the first months of pregnancy. The cardiovascular system is usually affected, in particular the tricuspid valve. A recent study has confirmed a 7% risk and given some valuable comparisons.[21] In a group of pregnant women suffering from manic depression the risk of fetal cardiac abnormalities was increased fivefold in those taking lithium compared with those taking other drugs. Nine out of 59 children born to mothers taking lithium were malformed or died soon after birth, compared with one of 38 taking drugs other than lithium.

Lithium clearance doubles during pregnancy, which may necessitate an increase in the patient's total daily intake of lithium to maintain the same serum concentration. At the time of delivery the clearance abruptly falls back to normal, and this may be sufficiently fast to precipitate toxic serum lithium concentrations in the mother. There is no evidence of a withdrawal reaction or behavioural abnormality in neonates exposed to lithium in utero.

Lithium enters the breast milk freely, and serum concentrations in neonates may be close to values that are therapeutic in adults.[22]

Toxicity may therefore supervene if there is negative sodium or water balance in the child. Lithium is therefore contraindicated for breast feeding mothers. Given the high risk of relapse of a biopolar illness in the puerperium, there are some unenviable choices to be made (see below). Carbamazepine is a possible alternative.

Anticonvulsants used in mood regulation

As a reaction to the need for regular estimations of serum concentrations and the risk of renal damage in long term treatment with lithium there has been a move towards using carbamazepine in both bipolar and unipolar manic-depressive illness. This is supported by well conducted double blind, placebo controlled trials. Rapid cycling disorder is considered to be a particular indication. Sodium valproate has also been proposed for use in this context.

Both carbamazepine and sodium valproate are clearly teratogenic. Carbamazepine exposure is associated with minor craniofacial defects, fingernail hypoplasia, and developmental delay[23], and there is a 1% risk of spina bifida. The causative agent may be the epoxide metabolite. Carbamazepine is excreted into breast milk, but low levels occur in the infant without observed toxicity. Sodium valproate is highly teratogenic; effects of its consumption during pregnancy include major and minor congenital abnormalities (neural tube defects and cleft palate), intrauterine growth retardation, hyperbilirubin anaemia, and potentially fatal hepatotoxicity. In breast feeding mothers, valproate gives rise to milk levels which are 15% of the maternal serum concentrations. No harmful effects on the nursing infant have been observed.

Guidelines for drug use during pregnancy and the puerperium

Patients already receiving treatment

The aim of minimising exposure of the fetus and the neonate to psychotropic drugs is helped enormously when patients are educated and enlightened about treatment. Lines of management differ for those known to have suffered a psychological disorder before the particular pregnancy and those whose illness has arisen for the first time during pregnancy or in the puerperium.

Patients already receiving long term psychotropic medication for psychosis should take contraceptive measures or, if no further children are wanted, should be offered sterilisation. The puerperium is a time of high risk of recurrence of a previous psychosis, with all that implies for the progression of secondary and tertiary handicap. This issue should be discussed with both the patient and her partner, not once but several times, in language that is clear and non-technical, to allow a satisfactory decision to be made. If such a patient is determined to conceive it will be a fine clinical decision whether to risk relapse by withdrawing psychotropic drugs or risk the slight possibility of fetal damage. The fetus may be harmed more by the effects of maternal relapse.

Lithium Patients receiving long term treatment with lithium are a particular problem if the question of another pregnancy is raised. A sudden desire for pregnancy may be a manifestation of a hypomanic mood swing, only partially controlled with the existing lithium carbonate treatment. Immediate withdrawl of lithium may result in a full blown illness. The issue must be discussed with the couple over several sessions, which will enable the would be mother's mental state to be more fully assessed. If lithium is to be withdrawn it should be done gradually over six or eight weeks to avoid a rebound relapse, and attempts at conception should be delayed to ensure that no recurrence of the illness follows in the weeks after treatment ends. The patient and her partner should be told that the risk of a peurperal psychosis may approach 1 in 5 if there was a previous non-puerperal manic-depressive episode. After a previous puerperal psychosis the risk is 1 in 5 for a manic illness and 1 in 10 for a psychotic depressive illness. For previous schizophrenic or atypical psychosis the risk is less.[4]

A patient who conceives while taking lithium or anticonvulsants and who presents wanting to continue the pregnancy should stop treatment immediately despite the risk of relapse. If further drug management is indicated on clinical grounds, neuroleptic drugs or tricyclic antidepressants should be prescribed. A pregnancy that has continued for some time with the mother taking lithium or anticonvulsants before its discovery is not an automatic indication for termination since the fetal cardiac abnormalities caused by this drug can usually be identified by ultrasound or amniotic fluid sampling.

In some patients, manic-depressive illnesses are so severe or difficult to treat, or adjustment is so precarious, that after the first trimester they will need to continue treatment with lithium or other neuroleptic maintenance treatment for the rest of the pregnancy. The serum lithium concentration should be maintained at a value as little above 0.5 mmol/1 at 12 hours after ingestion as possible. The daily lithium intake may need to be increased because of the change in the mother's lithium clearance. In these circumstances it is important that contact is established between the doctor monitoring treatment with lithium and other psychotropic drugs and the obstetrician. Obstetric management is easier if the mother is withdrawn gradually from her treatment in the weeks immediately before the estimated date of delivery.

Most puerperal psychoses start soon after delivery, and as withdrawal symptoms do not occur in neonates better protection is conferred by continuing lithium. Carbamazepine is an alternative if breast feeding is desired. The medical team has to decide which consideration is given priority.

A patient still receiving lithium treatment at term should be told to stop taking her tablets as soon as labour starts. No further lithium should be taken during labour, and fluid and electrolyte balance must be maintained. The serum lithium concentration must be monitored frequently, and diuretics should be avoided as they will delay lithium excretion.

Benzodiazepines Ideally, no patient should take benzodiazepines for more than five or six weeks, and even then they should be used on an "as needed" basis. Potential mothers who do use benzodiazepines regularly should be offered help with benzodiazepine withdrawal before conception takes place. Public awareness of the possible effects of drugs on the pregnancy and the fetus is increasing, but there is little point in inducing guilt and anxiety, which may put the benzodiazepine dependent mother in an impossible predicament. Women who have stopped taking benzodiazepines and who are having to cope with additional pressures of pregnancy will need extra support or even specific psychological treatment. This could be in a self help group or given individually by a community psychiatric nurse or health visitor.

Neuroleptic drugs Recent work suggests that many patients maintained on "standard" doses of depot neuroleptic drugs may do well with considerably lower doses and may need less additional treatment during any relapse. A pregnant patient who is receiving depot neuroleptic drugs may therefore have her regular dose reduced within the limitation of her clinical state. Depot neuroleptics take some time to clear after the last dose, which may have to be six or eight weeks before delivery is due so that the neonate is free from neuroleptic drugs.

Starting treatment in pregnancy

Treatment should not be skimped just because a patient is pregnant. For anxiety, intermittent use of benzodiazepines is preferable to day or night time exposure to retain the impact of the drug's action, to avoid dependence, and to minimise the effect on the fetus. Benzodiazepines with long half lives and active metabolites such as nitrazepam, diazepam, and chlordiazepoxide are best avoided in favour of drugs such as oxazepam. A major depressive illness with symptoms such as early morning wakening, diurnal variation, anorexia, poor concentration, guilt, and suicidal ideation may be treated in the normal way with tricyclic antidepressants if it occurs in pregnancy. If the depressive illness fails to respond to drug treatment electroconvulsive therapy may be used without harming the fetus or causing any long term damage. Electroconvulsive therapy is seldom necessary, but suicide in the context of a depressive illness in pregnancy is not unknown, and depressive illness at this time demands vigorous action. Without treatment, problems are likely to occur in the puerperium and afterwards.

Starting treatment in the puerperium

When a mother has had an episode of psychosis, whether in the puerperium or at another time, both she and her medical attendants will be concerned about the risk of recurrence. As the risk is about 20% and the interruption to mothering is so profound and long lasting, it is reasonable to offer such mothers prophylactic drug treatment immediately after delivery. Such a decision should be taken jointly by the general practitioner, obstetrician, and psychiatrist. The woman and her partner need to be fully informed and will want assurances about the effect that treatment will have on her and on her ability to look after the child and to breast feed. If the previous episode was a schizophrenic or depressive one, treatment with neuroleptic drugs or tricyclic antidepressants is straightforward and is compatible with breast feeding. Unless there is some guidance on dosage from the treatment of a previous episode, it may be necessary to start with small doses and to work up to chlorpromazine 150 mg a day or its equivalent. For tricylic antidepressants the dose is that required in treating a major depressive illness in a young adult: 100–150 mg amitriptyline or its equivalent a day. There is no reason to expect any untoward effects on the infant who is breast fed, but the health visitor has an important role in monitoring the child's progress.

In a patient with a history of biopolar manic-depressive illness, lithium is normally the drug of choices and breast feeding would be contraindicated. Serum concentrations should be monitored frequently to allow them to reach a full therapeutic value as soon as possible. Most postpartum psychiatric disorders occur within the first four or six weeks. If the mother seems normal at the end of this period the drug can be gradually withdrawn over the next month or two, but if there have been signs of a modified illness, treatment should be continued, with the same criteria as in episodes not occuring in the puerperium. The development of such an illness (albeit modified by prophylactic treatment) should be noted because it will have a bearing on the management of the patient after any subsequent pregnancy. Should the drug treatment fail to resolve the symptoms, further lines of treatment, including electroconvulsive therapy, should be used on the same basis as at any other time. A mother needs to be in as good a position as possible to care for her child, to maintain her marriage, and to have a satisfactory quality of life; the potential for suicide or infanticide in an untreated or partially treated psychotic mother adds emphasis to this point.

Key points

- Management differs for patients who had a psychiatric disorder before the pregnancy and those whose illness has arisen for the first time

- Treatment should not be skimped just because a patient is pregnant

- Withdrawing psychotropic medication in a patient determined to conceive may risk more harm to the fetus from the effects of maternal relapse than from the drug itself

- The risk of recurrence of psychosis is about 20%; mothers at risk should be offered prophylactic drug treatment immediately after delivery

PSYCHOTROPIC DRUGS

1 Kumar R, Robson K. A prospective study of emotional disorders in child bearing women. *B J Psychiatry* 1984; **144:** 35–47.
2 Cox J L, Connor Y, Kendell R E. Prospective study of the psychiatric disorders of childbirth by personal interview. *B J Psychiatry* 1982; **140:** 111–7.
3 Robin A A. Psychological changes of normal parturition. *Psychiatric Quarterly* 1962; **35:** 129–50.
4 Kendell R E, Chalmers J C, Platz C. The epidemiology of puerperal psychosis. *B J Psychiatry* 1987; **150:** 662–73.
5 Rosenberg L, Mitchell A A, Parsella J L, Parshayan H, Louick C, Shapiro S. Lack of relation of oral clefts to diazepam use during pregnancy. *N Engl J Med* 1983; **309:** 1282–5.
6 Bracken M B, Holford T R. Exposure to prescribed drugs in pregnancy and association with congenital malformations. *Obstet Gynaecol* 1981; **58:** 336–44.
7 Laegreid L, Olegard R, Walstrom J, Conradi N. Tetratogenic effects of benzodiazepine use during pregnancy. *J Paediat* 1989; **114:** 123–31.
8 Tyrer P, Owen R, Darling S. Gradual withdrawal of diazepam after long term therapy. *Lancet* 1983; i: 1402–6.
9 Kanto J H. The use of benzodiazepines during pregnancy labour and lactation with particular reference to pharmacokinetic considerations. 1982; **23:** 354–80.
10 Rementeria J L, Bhatt K. Withdrawal symptoms in neonates from intrauterine exposure to diazepam. 1977; **90:** 123–6.
11 Cree JE, Meyer J, Hailey DM. Diazepam in labour: its metabolism and effect on the clinical condition and thermogenesis of the newborn. *BMJ* 1973; iv: 251–5.
12 Tomson G, Lunnell N O. Transplacental passage and kinetics in the mother and newborn of oxazepam giving during labour. *Clin Pharmacol Therapeut* 1979; **25:** 74–81.
13 Rieder R D. The offspring of schizophrenics — fetal and neonatal death. *Arch Gen Psychiatry* 1975; **32:** 200–11.
14 Ananth J. Congenital malformations with psychopharmacologic agents. *Compr Psychiatry* 1975; **16:** 437–45.
15 Schrire I. Trifluoperazine and foetal abnormalities. *Lancet* 1963; i: 174.
16 Hill R M, Desmond M M, Kay J I. Extrapyramidal dysfunction in an infant of a schizophrenic mother. *J Paediat* 1966; **69:** 589–95.
17 Webster P A. Withdrawal symptoms in neonates associated with maternal antidepressant therapy. *Lancet* 1973; ii: 318–9.
18 Heinonen P, Slone D, Shapiro S. *Birth defects and drugs in pregnancy*. Littleton, MA: Publishing Sciences Group, 1977: 336–7.
19 Ayd FJ Jr. Children born of mothers treated with chlorpromazine during pregnancy. *Clin Med* 1964; **71:** 1758–63.
20 Takyo B E. Excretion of drugs in human milk. *Am J Hosp Pharm* 1970; **28:** 317–26.
21 Kallen B, Tandbery A. Lithium and pregnancy — a cohort study on manic depressive women. *Acta Psychiat Scand* 1983; **68:** 134–9.
22 Schon M, Amdisen A. Lithium and pregnancy. III. Lithium ingestion by children breast fed by women on lithium treatment. *BMJ* 1973; iii: 138.
23 Jones K L, Lacro R V, Johnson K A, Adams J. Teratogenic effects of carbamezepine. *J Med* 1989; **321:** 1481.

8 Treatment of endocrine diseases

WM HAGUE

This chapter reviews the use of drugs in pregnancy in all the main areas of endocrine disorder except diabetes mellitus, which is dealt with separately.

Drugs are used for both diagnosis and management of endocrine diseases. Diagnosis involves assessment of basal function of an endocrine gland, followed by tests to suppress or stimulate that gland. Further diagnostic measures may well include localisation procedures. Medical management usually consists of hormone replacement therapy when there is endocrine failure, or suppressive treatment in the case of hyperfunction.

Diagnostic measures

Pregnancy usually requires a state of endocrine balance; the changes of conception are reduced unless the endocrine milieu is normal. Endocrine disease does, however, arise de novo in both pregnancy and the puerperium. This section deals with tests of endocrine function that require the use of drugs: the diagnosis of thyrotoxicosis and, less commonly, the adrenal disorders that cause hypertension and pituitary disease.

Thyrotoxicosis

After diabetes, thyrotoxicosis is the most common endocrine problem developing in pregnancy; many of the signs mimic those of normal pregnancy. Diagnosis depends on the measurement of pituitary thyrotrophin, which is suppressed in active disease. The introduction of the sensitive radio-immunometric assay (IRMA) for thyrotrophin has now almost done away with the need for the thyrotrophin releasing hormone test in the assessment of thyroid function as a measure of pituitary thyrotrophin response. Doubts have been expressed about the use of thyrotrophin in early pregnancy because of its effect of producing smooth muscle contraction.[1] It may also exacerbate hypertension.[2] Another diagnostic measure in thyrotoxicosis, measurement of iodine-131 uptake, is totally contraindicated in ongoing pregnancy because of the risk of fetal uptake of the isotope and subsequent thyroidal damage, although complete destruction of the thyroid has not been documented with the diagnostic dose.[3]

Adrenal disorders that cause hypertension

Phaeochromocytoma may be suspected with raised excretion of catecholamines or their metabolites. Pentolinium, a quaternary ammonium ganglion blocking compound, has been used as a diagnostic agent. Failure to reduce plasma catecholamine concentrations after intravenous injection of pentolinium 5 mg provides additional evidence for establishing the diagnosis,[4] but no experience of this test in pregnancy has been described. Localisation procedures for phaeochromocytoma include the use of [^{131}I]-met-iodobenzylguanidine: this should be avoided in pregnancy because of the radiation risk to the fetal thyroid.

Conn's syndrome – Mineralocorticoid excess is rare but may be suspected in patients with hypertension and hypokalaemia. The hypertension is rarely severe, and full investigation may be postponed until after pregnancy, when localisation procedures, such as the use of radiolabelled selenium cholesterol, may be used without fear of fetal compromise.

Cushing's syndrome – Though rare, glucocorticoid excess presenting in pregnancy is serious and needs urgent investigation because of the high risk (10%) of malignancy of the adrenal cortex.[5] Dexamethasone crosses the placenta with suppression of the fetal pituitary-adrenal axis,[6] but in the doses used for diagnosis this suppression is short lived. The use of metyrapone is discussed in the section on management.

Pituitary disorders

Investigation of pituitary disease usually includes assessing the response to insulin induced hypoglycaemia. The transient nature of the hypoglycaemia is without serious risk to the fetus. The usual precautions of having an intravenous line open, with hydrocortisone and dextrose drawn up ready, as well as using a smaller dose of insulin for patients suspected of hypopituitarism, apply in pregnancy as much as for the non-pregnant patient.

Management: hormone replacement therapy

Hypothyroidism

Hypothyroidism is usually diagnosed and treated before pregnancy, as the hypothyroid state is often associated with infertility. There is also a high risk of poor pregnancy outcome, before thyroid replacement, including frequent spontaneous abortions, a doubled stillbirth rate, an increased incidence of premature labour, and subnormal neonatal neurological development.[7] An increased risk of congenital abnormality in the offspring of these patients has been questioned.[8] Thyroid replacement is achieved with L-thyroxine 100–200 μg a day as a single dose, monitoring response by the fall of the serum TSH concentration. In pregnancy the dose of thyroxine can usually be maintained.[9] The important point is to monitor and treat according to the results of biochemistry rather than by clinical judgment. Testing thyroid function once in each trimester is usually sufficient. In the puerperium, any increase in thyroxine dose will need reduction again. There is no contraindication to breast feeding.

Hypoadrenalism

As with hypothyroidism, adrenal insufficiency is usually diagnosed and treated before pregnancy is possible. Replacement therapy (hydrocortisone 20–30 mg a day, fludrocortisone 0.05–0.20 mg a day) is essential, but needs no alteration in pregnancy unless intercurrent stress or illness occurs, when increased or parenteral doses should be used. The oestrogen mediated rise in cortisol binding globulin during pregnancy does not seem to affect steroid requirements. There may be an increased incidence of infants small for gestational age in Addison's disease[10]; it is not clear whether this is due to the disease or the treatment. No other complication, either fetal or maternal, has been associated with steroid replacement therapy. Breast feeding is not a problem.

Hypopituitarism

Anterior pituitary deficiency states require thyroxine and corticosteroid replacement as above, with the exception that fludrocortisone is not required as mineralocorticoid secretion is independent of the pituitary. Untreated, hypopituitarism has a high mortality for both fetus and mother.[11] Hypogonadotrophic states may require exogenous gonadotrophin or, more physiologically, pulsatile gonadotrophin releasing hormone, for ovulation to occur. Once pregnancy is achieved, however, maintenance therapy is not necessary because of the gonadotrophin and sex steroid production by the fetoplacental unit. Lactation may be impaired because of prolactin deficiency.

Posterior pituitary failure is associated with diabetes insipidus, requiring the use of the vasopressin analogue desmopressin (DDAVP) (5–10 μg twice a day) as replacement. A review of 67 cases showed that 58% of patients showed deterioration during pregnancy.[12] The mechanism for this is unclear but may reflect the increase in metabolic clearance of vasopressin in pregnancy. No ill effects of desmopressin in pregnancy have been reported apart from a small risk of increased uterine contractility due to the oxytocin-like structure and activity of the drug.[13] This effect is seen when desmopressin is used intravenously as a diagnostic agent rather than with the normal replacement regimen using nasal insufflation. Desmopressin has 75 times less oxytocic action than arginine vasopressin.

Hypoparathyroidism

Usually associated with the post-thyroidectomy state, but occasionally seen as part of an autoimmune diathesis or as a hormone resistant syndrome, hypoparathyroidism in the mother poses severe risks of fetal hyperparathyroidism with neonatal hypocalcaemic rickets that may be fatal. Treatment with calcium (1600–2000 μg a day) and either vitamin D (1·25–2·5 mg a day) or dihydrotachysterol (250–1000 μg a day) is essential, with frequent monitoring of maternal serum Ca^{2+} and PO_4^{2-} to maintain normocalcaemia.[14] The vitamin D requirement increases twofold to threefold during pregnancy.[15] The use of calcitriol has been associated with fetal hypermineralisation in one of twin fetuses.[16]

In the puerperium, the requirement for calcium and vitamin D·
should be reassessed without delay; they may not be required at
all.[17] In the normal woman, an insignificant amount of vitamin D
is secreted in the breast milk,[18] but the high doses of vitamin D
required in lactating hypoparathyroid women may cause neonatal
hypervitaminosis.

Ovarian failure

For many years, the prospect of pregnancy in the patient with
ovarian failure seemed remote, but oocyte donation, in vitro
fertilisation, and embryo transfer have made this a possibility.
Patient preparation includes the use of oestrogen and progesterone to prepare the recipient uterus and endometrium before
embryo transfer and subsequently to maintain the hormonal
environment until the fetoplacental unit can take over. The use of
sex steroids in pregnancy is discussed below.

Management: endocrine gland hyperfunction

Thyrotoxicosis

The mainstays of medical treatment of thyrotoxicosis are the
thionamide agents: carbimazole, propylthiouracil, and, less
commonly used in Britain and Australasia, methimazole.
Prophylthiouracil is less lipid soluble and more highly protein
bound than carbimazole or methimazole and is less readily
transferred into the breast milk[19] or, theoretically, across the
placenta. No teratogenic effects have been reported for
prophylthiouracil or carbimazole, but there have been five cases
of a scalp defect, aplasia cutis, occurring in neonates whose
mothers had been treated with methimazole.[20] One study
suggested that maternal thyrotoxicosis may itself be associated
with fetal malformation, and that the risk may be reduced by
antithyroid drug treatment.[21] Perinatal mortality is also high in
untreated thyrotoxicosis, with a high incidence of premature
delivery that can be reduced to normal with treatment.[22] Fetal
hypothyroidism is a definite risk with all thionamide treatment,
and the lowest possible dose to maintain biochemical euthyroid-
ism in the mother must be used, with (at least) monthly checks on
the free thyroid hormone and thyrotrophin concentrations. Fetal
goitre formation, however, is not dose related and is also affected
by maternal antibody status and iodine intake. The intellectual

development of children exposed to antithyroid drugs in utero is reported to be unaffected.[22] Autoimmune thyrotoxicosis often improves during pregnancy so that dosage of antithyroid drugs may be reduced, but after delivery a flare of overactivity is common,[23] requiring an increase in treatment.

Other agents used to control thyrotoxicosis include β blocking drugs, potassium iodide, and radioactive iodine. (For a full discussion of β blockade, see chapter 9 on cardiovascular disease.) Potassium iodide, often used in preparation for thyroid surgery, is well recognised as a cause of fetal goitre[24]; cases of fetal goitre have been reported when the mother took as little as 12 mg iodide a day. Radioactive iodine (^{131}I) in therapeutic doses is liable to ablate the fetal thyroid and also has the potential to induce maternal thyroid storm (see below). Paradoxically, the risk to the fetus is least in the first trimester, before the fetal iodine trap is operational.[25]

In the light of the above, propylthiouracil is probably the drug of choice in both pregnancy and puerperium. Initially 100–150 mg should be taken every 8 hours, and this should be reduced to 50 mg every 6–8 hours once the hyperthyroid state is controlled clinically and, more importantly, biochemically. The lowest possible maintenance dose should be used to maintain the serum free thyroxine concentration in the high normal range. If thyrotoxicosis recurs or is not controlled, up to 600 mg a day in divided doses may be used. Failure to control symptoms may indicate the need for partial thyroidectomy, in which case propranolol (40 mg every 6 hours) may be given to control residual symptoms before surgery.

Fetal and neonatal thyrotoxicosis may occur as a result of the transplacental passage of thyroid stimulating antibodies in the absence of maternal signs after thyroid ablation or, rarely, in maternal autoimmune hypothyroidism. Thionamides have been used successfully to control the fetal thyrotoxicosis, with the fetal heart rate being monitored as a guide to dose.[26] Intra-amniotic administration of thyroxine has been used in a case of suspected fetal hypothyroidism,[27] but experience with this is limited and careful follow up of such infants is needed.

In unrecognised thyrotoxicosis the stress of an infection or labour or operative delivery may lead to the onset of thyroid storm. Though rare, this is a medical emergency with a high risk of morbidity and mortality to mother and fetus. Intravenous fluids, high doses of propylthiuracil (600–800 mg immediately,

150–200 mg 4–6 hourly) ,followed one to two hours later by iodide therapy (potassium iodide 2–5 drops by mouth, or sodium iodide 0·5–1·0 g intravenously, every 8 hours), dexamethasone (2 mg 6 hourly, given four times), propranolol (20–80 mg by mouth or 1–10 mg intravenously, every 4 hours), phenobarbitone (30–60 mg 6–8 hourly), oxygen and supportive therapy should be given, preferably in an intensive care or high dependency setting.[28] Treatment should be started without waiting for laboratory confirmation of hyperthyroidism.

Cushing's syndrome

Drugs used in the management of Cushing's syndrome include metyrapone, trilostane, and aminoglutethimide, all of which block various points in the biosynthetic pathway of cortisol, and cyproheptadine, a serotonin antagonist which is used to suppress corticotrophin releasing hormone. Experience of the use of all these drugs in pregnancy is limited because of the rarity of the syndrome. Metyrapone has not been shown to have any adverse effects on fetus or mother in normal pregnancy.[29] Studies in baboons have shown an inhibition of surfactant release, but the offspring did not develop respiratory distress.[30] Metyrapone has been used successfully in Cushing's syndrome in pregnancy, with survival of both mother and infant,[31] but in a second report the use of metyrapone coincided with the onset of severe pre-eclampsia at just over 26 weeks' gestation, and the infant died as a result of premature delivery.[32] The link between the use of metyrapone, which increases 11-deoxycorticosterone production, and the exacerbation of maternal hypertension in this case is not clear. Trilostane, which antagonises 3βOH-steroid dehydrogenase, inhibits placental progesterone production, with the risk of abortion or premature labour,[33] and is therefore contraindicated in pregnancy. The use of aminoglutethimide and cyproheptadine has been reported in one case each, but with limited data as to outcome.[34,35]

In view of the high proportion (10%) of adrenal malignancy among pregnant patients with Cushing's syndrome, active surgical or obstetric management, or both, has been recommended in the first and last trimesters; metyrapone should be reserved for the difficult problems of the second trimester.[36] There are no data on the use of metyrapone in lactating women; it is lipid soluble and therefore likely to be excreted into the breast milk.

Congenital adrenal hyperplasia

Adrenal suppression in patients with congenital adrenal hyperplasia is achieved with replacement glucocorticoid and mineralocorticoid therapy, which should be maintained in pregnancy as for patients with hypoadrenalism (see above). The fetus with adrenal hyperplasia has been treated by giving dexamethasone to the mother in the first and second trimesters to suppress fetal production of adrenocorticotrophic hormone, thus reducing fetal adrenal androgen output with its associated masculinisation of female genitalia.[37] Risks to the mother of this treatment include hypertension, diabetes, and osteoporosis.

Phaeochromocytoma

The management of phaeochromocytoma in pregnancy is surgical, once control of the circulating catecholamine effects has been achieved with the use of α and β adrenoceptor blocking agents.

Hyperprolactinaemia and acromegaly

The dopaminergic agent bromocriptine is the drug of choice in the management of hyperprolactinaemia caused by pituitary microadenomata or macroadenomata; it allows ovulation and reduces tumour size. It has a place in the management of acromegaly as it reduces growth hormone secretion, although this is not always so successful. It has been used to suppress lactation, but concern over the increased risk of cerebrovascular accidents,[38] particularly in women with hypertension or pre-eclampsia, has resulted in the product licence for this indication being withdrawn in Australia and the United States. No ill effects to the fetus have been reported, either in women in whom ovulation was induced with bromocriptine or in women given bromocriptine throughout pregnancy,[39] although there is evidence that bromocriptine, or an active metabolite, does cross the placenta.[40]

The use of bromocriptine in pregnancy should be reserved for the small number of women who present with symptoms and signs of tumour expansion, in whom high resolution computed tomography or magnetic resonance imaging confirms the diagnosis, and in whom immediate delivery is not practicable or desirable.[41] Treatment starts at 5 mg a day in divided doses, doubling daily over 3 days until symptoms resolve or the patient is taking 20 mg a day or has developed side effects. Surgery is rarely necessary. Lactation in such patients is both suppressed and contraindicated, and early contraception must be considered.

The use of the somatostatin analogue octreotide in pregnancy has not been reported.

Hyperparathyroidism

The treatment of symptomatic hyperparathyroidism in pregnancy is surgical. Fluid replacement may be necessary before operation if the hypercalcaemia is severe.[42] Mild hypercalcaemia without symptoms may respond to phosphate or magnesium. The neonate needs careful observation for signs of hypocalcaemia (secondary to parathormone suppression), which may present late in the postnatal period.

Sex hormones and pregnancy

Oestrogen containing compounds are commonly used to inhibit ovulation and thus avoid pregnancy. In practice, pregnancy has often occurred while oestrogen was taken because of impaired absorption or a missed pill or too low a dose. Oestrogens have also been used to inhibit lactation. Non-steroidal oestrogens, such as stilboestrol, hexoestrol, and dienoestrol, have been clearly shown to be teratogenic, and the association with adenocarcinoma of the vagina and cervix in female offspring of mothers treated before the 18th week of gestation is well documented.[43] Other changes of the female genital tract have occurred, and male offspring of such mothers have been found to have testicular, seminal, and other genital abnormalities.[44]

Steroidal oestrogens do not have the same effects as the stilboestrol-like compounds,[43] but there is disagreement about their teratogenicity, in particular whether they are associated with anomalies of the cardiovascular system, limb deformities, neural tube defects, and renal and tracheo-oesophageal abnormalities.[45] Two large prospective studies found no increased risk to babies born to mothers who conceived either after or while taking oral contraception.[46,47]

Many of the progestagens used as contraceptive agents, such as norethisterone and levonorgestrel, are 19-nortestosterone derivatives with mildly androgenic properties and could cause virilisation of a female fetus, although the small amounts present in oral contraceptives are unlikely to do so. 17-Hydroxyprogesterone derivatives such as medroxyprogesterone acetate (Provera) and 17-hydroxyprogesterone caproate (Proluton) are pure progestational compounds and have been used in the management of habitual abortion, although their use is now controversial.[48]

The weak androgen danazol has been used in the treatment of endometriosis to suppress ovarian activity and menstruation. Ovulation does occasionally occur at low doses, and danazol has been associated with masculinisation of a female fetus.[49] The manufacturers recommend the use of concurrent non-hormonal contraception.

The antiandrogen cyproterone acetate has been shown to inhibit masculinisation of the male fetus in animal studies,[50] and is recommended in combination with oestrogen to provide contraception as well as to enhance the antiandrogenic effects. No such effects have been reported in the fetuses of women treated with the low dose of cyproterone acetate as found in Diane-35.

The anti-oestrogen clomiphene citrate has been implicated in several case reports of neural tube defects. Large studies have not, however, shown any significant increase in the malformation rate.[51]

The use of sex steroids in lactating women deserves comment. The use of high dose oestrogen to suppress lactation has for long been considered a risk because of thromboembolism.[52] Because the risk of venous thromboembolism is greatest after delivery, it is wise to avoid compounds containing oestrogen in the immediate and early puerperium. Progestagen-only contraception is preferable as it has no effect on lactation or coagulation.[53] If the milk supply is diminishing or needs supplementation, or when menses return, a transfer to a combined preparation is recommended if maximum effectiveness is required. Cyproterone acetate is contraindicated until weaning is complete as there is a definite risk of transfer in the breast milk,[54] although the effects on the neonate are not known.

Key points

- Thyroid replacement should be monitored by measurement of thyrotrophin once in each trimester
- Antithyroid drugs should be used in the lowest dose which keeps the mother euthyroid
- Oral contraceptives do not seem to be teratogenic
- Oral contraceptives containing oestrogen should be avoided in the early puerperium because of thromboembolic risk and possible reduction in milk supply

1 Reynolds JEF, ed. *Martindale: The extra pharmacopoeia.* London: Pharmaceutical Press, 1982: 1276–7.

2 Borowski GD, Garofano CD, Rose LI, Levy RA. Blood pressure response to thyrotropin releasing hormone in euthyroid subjects. *J Clin Endocrinol Metab* 1984; **38**: 197–202

3 Hays PM, Cruikshank DP. Hormonal therapy during pregnancy. In: Eskes TKAB, Finster M, eds, *Drug therapy during pregnancy.* London: Butterworth, 1985: 110–60.

4 Brown MJ, Allison DJ, Jenner DA, Lewis PJ, Dollery CT. Increased sensitivity and accuracy of phaeochromocytoma diagnosis achieved by use of plasma-adrenaline estimations and a pentolinium-suppression test. *Lancet* 1981; i: 174–7.

5 Buescher MA, McClamrock HD, Adashi EY. Cushing syndrome in pregnancy. *Obstet Gynecol* 1992; **79**: 130–7.

6 Funkhouser JD, Peery KJ, Mockridge PB, Hughes ER. Distribution of dexamethasone between mother and fetus after maternal administration. *Pediatr Res* 1978; **12**: 1053–6.

7 Thomas R, Reid RL. Thyroid disease and reproductive dysfunction. *Obstet Gynecol* 1987; **70**: 789–98.

8 Montoro M, Collea JV, Frasier SN, Mestman JH. Successful outcome of pregnancy in women with hypothyroidism. *Ann Intern Med* 1981; **94**: 31–4.

9 Girling JC, de Swiet M. Thyroxine dosage during pregnancy in women with primary hypothyroidism. *Br J Obstet Gynaecol* 1992; **99**: 368–70.

10 Osler M. Addison's disease and pregnancy. *Acta Endocrinol* 1962; **41**: 67–78.

11 Grimes HG, Brooks MH. Pregnancy in Sheehan's syndrome. Report of a case and review. *Obstet Gynecol Surv* 1980; **35**: 481–8.

12 Hime MC, Richardson JA. Diabetes insipidus and pregnancy. Case report, incidence, and review of the literature. *Obstet Gynecol Surv* 1978; **33**: 375–9.

13 Baylis PH, Thompson C, Burd J, Tunbridge WM, Snodgrass CA. Recurrent pregnancy induced polyuria and thirst due to hypothalamic diabetes insipidus: an investigation into possible mechanisms responsible for polyuria. *Clin Endocrinol* 1986; **24**: 459–66.

14 Montoro M, Mestman JH. How to manage parathyroid disease in the pregnant patient and neonate. *Contemporary Obstetrics and Gynaecology* 1981; **17**: 143–57.

15 Sadeghi-Nejad A, Wolfsdorg JI, Senior B. Hypoparathyroidism and pregnancy treatment with calcitriol. *JAMA* 1980; **243**: 254–5.

16 Salle BL, Berthezene F, Glorieux FH, Delvin EE, Berland M, David L, *et al.* Hypoparathyroidism during pregnancy: treatment with calcitriol. *J Clin Endocrinol Metab* 1981; **52**: 810–3.

17 Wright AD, Joplin GF, Dixon HG. Post-partum hypercalcaemia in treated hypoparathyroidism. *BMJ* 1969; i: 23–5.

18 Beeley L. Drugs and breastfeeding. *Clin Obstet Gynaecol* 1986; **13**: 247–51.

19 Kampmann JP, Hansen JM, Johansen K, Helweg J. Propylthiouracil in human milk. *Lancet* 1980; i: 736–7.

20 Mujtaba Q, Burrow GN. Treatment of hyperthyroidism in pregnancy with propylthiouracil and methimazole. *Obstet Gynecol* 1975; **46**: 282–6.

21 Momotani M, Ito K, Hamada N, Ban Y, Nishikawa Y, Mimura T. Maternal hyperthyroidism and congenital malformation in the offspring. *Clin Endocrinol* 1984; **20**: 695–700.

22 Burrow GN, Bartsocas D, Klatskin DH, Grunt JA. Children exposed in utero to propylthiouracil. *Am J Dis Child* 1968; **116**: 161–5.

23 Amino N, Miyai K, Yamamoto T, Kuro T, Tanaka F, Tanizawa O, *et al.* Transient recurrence of hyperthyroidism after delivery in Graves' disease. *J Clin Endocrinol Metab* 1977; **44**: 130–6.

24 Senior B, Chernoff HL. Iodide goiter in the newborn. *Pediatrics* 1971; **47**: 510–5.

25 Stouffer SS, Hamburger JT. Inadvertent ^{131}I therapy for hyperthyroidism in the first trimester of pregnancy. *J Nucl Med* 1976; **17**: 146–9.

26 Cove DH, Johnston P. Fetal hyperthyroidism: experience of treatment in four siblings. *Lancet* 1985; i: 430–2.

27 Lightner ES, Fismer DA, Giles H, Woolfenden J. Intra-amniotic injection of thyroxine (T4) to a human fetus. *Am J Obstet Gynecol* 1977; **127**: 487–90.

28 Molitch M. Endocrine emergencies in pregnancy. *Baillière's Clin Endocrinol Metab* 1992; **6**: 167–91.

29 Heinen G, Buchheit M, Oertal W. Untersuchungen mit dem Adrenostatikum SU4885 (Metopiron) in der Schwangerschaft. *Klin Wochensch* 1963; **41**: 103–5.

30 Kling OR, Kotas RV. Endocrine influences on pulmonary maturation and the lecithin/sphingomyelin ratio in the fetal baboon. *Am J Obstet Gynecol* 1975; **121**: 664–8.

31 Gormley MJJ, Hadden DR, Kennedy TL, Montgomery DAD, Murnaghan GA, Sheridan

    B. Cushing's syndrome in pregnancy – treatment with metyrapone. *Clin Endocrinol* 1982; **16**: 283–93.

32 Connell JMC, Cordiner J, Davies DL, Fraser R, Frier BM, McPherson SG. Pregnancy complicated by Cushing's syndrome: potential hazard of metyrapone therapy. Case report. *Br J Obstet Gynaecol* 1985; **92**: 1192–5.

33 Van der Spuy ZM, Jones DL, Wright CSW, Piura B, Paintin DB, James VHT, *et al.* Inhibition of 3β hydroxysteroid dehydrogenase activity in first trimester human pregnancy with trilostane and WIN 32729. *Clin Endocrinol* 1983; **19**: 521–2.

34 Hanson TJ, Ballonoff LB, Northcutt RC. Aminoglutethimide and pregnancy. *JAMA* 1974; **230**: 963–4.

35 Aron DC, Schall AM, Sheeler LR. Cushing's syndrome and pregnancy. *Am J Obstet Gynecol* 1990; **162**: 244–52.

36 Van der Spuy ZM, Jacobs HS. Management of endocrine disorders in pregnancy - part II. *Postgrad Med J* 1984; **60**: 312–20.

37 Forest MG, David M, Morel Y. Prenatal diagnosis and treatment of 21-hydroxylase deficiency. *J Steroid Biochem Mol Biol* 1993; **45**: 75–82.

38 Kulig K, Moore LL, Kirk M, Smith D, Stallworth J, Berwick B. Bromocryptine-associated headache: possible life-threatening sympathomimetic interaction. *Obstet Gynecol* 1991; **78**: 941–3.

39 Krupp P, Turkalj I. Surveillance of Parlodel (bromocriptine) in pregnancy and offspring. In: Jacobs HS, ed. *Prolactinomas and pregnancy*. Lancaster: MTP Press, 1984: 45–50.

40 Bigazzi M, Ronga R, Lancranjan I, Ferraro S, Branconi F, Buzzoni P, *et al.* A pregnancy in an acromegalic woman during bromocryptine treatment: effects on growth hormone and prolactin in the maternal, fetal and amniotic compartments. *J Clin Endocrinol Metab* 1979; **48**: 9–12.

41 Bergh T, Nillius SJ. Prolactinomas in pregnancy. In: Jacobs HS, ed. *Prolactinomas and pregnancy*. Lancaster: MTP Press, 1984: 41–5.

42 Clark D, Seeds JW, Cefalo RC. Hyperparathyroid crisis and pregnancy. *Am J Obstet Gynecol* 1981; **140**: 840–2.

43 Herbst AL, Kurman RJ, Scully RE, Poskanzer DC. Clear-cell adenocarcinoma of the genital tract in young females: registry report. *N Eng J Med* 1972; **287**: 1259–64.

44 Stillman RJ. In utero exposure to diethylstilboestrol: adverse effects on the reproductive tract and reproductive performance in male and female offspring. *Am J Obstet Gynecol* 1982; **142**: 905–21.

45 Wilson JG, Brent RL. Are female sex hormones teratogenic? *Am J Obstet Gynecol* 1981; **141**: 567–80.

46 Royal College of General Practitioners' Oral Contraception Study. The outcome of pregnancy in former oral contraceptive users. *Br J Obstet Gynaecol* 1976; **83**: 608–16.

47 Vessey M, Meisler L, Flavel R, Yeates D. Outcome of pregnancy in women using different methods of contraception. *Br J Obstet Gynaecol* 1979; **86**: 548–56.

48 MacDonald RR. Does treatment with progesterone prevent miscarriage? *Br J Obstet Gynaecol* 1989; **96**: 257–64.

49 Shaw RW, Farquhar JW. Female pseudohermaphroditism associated with danazol exposure in utero. Case report. *Br J Obstet Gynaecol* 1984; **91**: 386–9.

50 Hamada H, Neumann F, Junkmann K. Intrauterine antimaskuline Beeinflussung von Rattenfeten durch ein stark gestagen wirksames Steroid. *Acta Endocrinol* 1963; **44**: 380–8.

51 Kurachi K, Aono T, Minigawa J, Miyake A. Congenital malformations of newborn infants after clomiphene-induced ovulation. *Fertil Steril* 1983; **40**: 187–9.

52 Daniel DG, Campbell H, Turnbull AC. Puerperal thromboembolism and suppression of lactation. *Lancet* 1967; **ii**: 287–9.

53 Guillebaud J. Combined oral contraceptive pills. In: Loudon N, ed. *Handbook of family planning*. Edinburgh: Churchill Livingstone, 1991: 63–124.

54 Stoppelli I, Rainer E, Humpel M. Transfer of cyproterone acetate to the milk of lactating women. *Contraception* 1980; **22**: 485–93.

9 Treatment of cardiovascular diseases

HELEN E HOPKINSON

Pregnant women may require drug treatment for chronic cardiovascular disease which antedates the pregnancy or for disease which develops or merits treatment for the first time in pregnancy. Broadly speaking, the disorder will be either hypertension or a dysrrhythmia. Heart failure is rare in pregnancy and requires specialist assessment and management beyond the scope of this chapter.

Essential hypertension

Young patients with essential hypertension are often prescribed an angiotension converting enzyme inhibitor once daily for ease of compliance and because there are few side effects. This is especially so in diabetic patients with microalbuminuria or nephropathy, in whom angiotension converting enzyme inhibitors provide an additional renoprotective effect. These drugs are contraindicated in pregnancy: intrauterine death in animal studies[1] and oligohydramnios, fetal anuria, and stillbirth in humans later in pregnancy have been reported.[2–7] Captopril and enalapril limited to the first trimester do not seem to present a significant risk to the fetus. Nevertheless, women taking angiotension converting enzyme inhibitors who are contemplating pregnancy should be changed to one of the alternatives below which have been more fully evaluated.

Hypertension developing in pregnancy

Several antihypertensive agents are safe and effective both in pregnancy induced hypertension and in pre-eclampsia. The purpose of treatment remains to protect the mother from disasters such as intracerebral haemorrhage, but the prescriber's concern (and usually the mother's) is to ensure fetal well being.

Drugs suitable for outpatient treatment or non-urgent blood pressure control

Methyldopa is regarded as a safe antihypertensive drug for use throughout pregnancy.[8] It crosses the placenta and is found in cord blood at a similar concentration to that in the mother.[9] It reduces systolic blood pressure in neonates,[10] but there have been no reports of adverse fetal effects. Data for over seven years of paediatric follow up of infants whose mothers were treated in pregnancy with methyldopa for hypertension or pre-eclampsia show no evidence of any long term abnormalities in infant development.[11]

Maternal side effects of methyldopa are manifestations of the drug's central nervous depressant action and include drowsiness, depression, and postural hypotension. These may result in treatment being stopped in some individuals. Despite this, methyldopa remains a first line drug for essential hypertension in the months before conception and for antihypertensive treatment started during pregnancy.

β Adrenergic blocking agents are widely used in pregnancy for treating hypertension. They are effective, and many have been evaluated in clinical trials, although only two such trials had placebo controls.[12,13] Early anecdotal and retrospective reports of fetal complications and death due to propranolol were not confirmed in prospective controlled studies. β Blockers cross the placenta and may cause a harmless lowering of fetal heart rate, but cardiotocographic reactivity is not affected.[14] If treatment with atenolol is started before 28 weeks' gestation, gestationally adjusted birthweight is reduced,[15] but there is no evidence of persistent effects on infant growth.[16] Reported effects on fetal growth vary between different β blockers, and there is inconsistency between different trials using the same drug.[17–19] However, prolonged treatment with methyldopa started before 28 weeks did not decrease birth weight in comparison with untreated controls.[8]

Maternal benefits in addition to the antihypertensive effect have been documented, though again the results of trials are conflicting. Treatment with atenolol,[12] acebutolol,[20] and labetalol[21-23] has been associated with a decreased incidence of proteinuria later on, and even an improvement of pre-existing proteinuria. β Blockers are better tolerated than methyldopa, and a placebo controlled, double blind trial of atenolol showed no difference between the treatment groups in maternal symptoms that could have been attributed to β blockers.[12]

In summary, β blockers are safe antihypertensive agents for use in the third trimester. Though no single β blocker has been shown to be superior; if treatment is to be started before 28 weeks methyldopa should be the first choice.

Calcium channel antagonists – namely nifedipine, nicardipine, and nitrendipine – have been shown to decrease blood pressure in pregnancy[24-26] and to control antenatal and postpartum hypertension.[27] No controlled studies of long term treatment or assessment of fetal risk have been reported. In acute severe hypertension nifedipine can be given orally or sublingually as an alternative to a parenteral drug; it has a relatively quick onset of action. These drugs also have tocolytic activity, through relaxation of uterine smooth muscle, and nifedipine has been used for this purpose in premature labour in normotensive women.[24]

Maternal side effects include facial flushing, headache, and oedema, which can be so great as to require discontinuing the drug.

Diuretic agents are effective antihypertensives that are widely prescribed in the general population. They reduce effective circulating volume, which is theoretically disadvantageous in women with hypertensive disease in pregnancy as their intravascular volume may already be reduced.[28] Further depletion may seriously compromise uteroplacental blood flow, which in many cases will already be impaired. An overview of the use of mainly thiazide diuretics in pregnancy, however, showed no adverse fetal effects.[29] In practice, in the antenatal clinic diuretics are not used for hypertensive diseases or simple oedema but are reserved for treating heart failure.

Prasozin is an α adrenoreceptor blocker that has been used in pregnancy as second line antihypertensive treatment, usually in combination with a β blocking agent. Such a regimen led to improved blood pressure control in severe hypertension when prasozin was used with oxprenolol.[30] Fetal malformation has not been reported although most experience is of its use later in pregnancy. The bioavailability of prasozin is increased during pregnancy[31] so small doses (0·5 mg) should be used, and appropriate precautions should be taken against first dose hypotension.

Hydralazine is another vasodilator that is an effective second line antihypertensive when it is used in conjunction with methyldopa or β blockers. Maternal compensatory tachycardia can be controlled with β blockade, but headache and facial flushing are less well tolerated. There are rare reports of neuropathy and lupus-like syndromes associated with hydralazine. Fetal problems are also rare, but neonatal thrombocytopaenia has been recorded and linked to the use of hydralazine in the mother.

Drugs for hypertensive emergencies

The treatment for uncontrolled hypertension and pre-eclampsia is delivery. Nevertheless, blood pressure must be controlled in labour or before anaesthesia. Ultimately an epidural anaesthetic is useful in this context, but according to the condition of the patient either quick acting oral or parenteral drugs will be required.

Nifedipine has already been described. It is absorbed readily via the sublingual route in acute severe hypertension.

Hydralazine can be administered parenterally but it takes 20–30 minutes to act. The maternal side effects may interfere with interpretation of the patient's condition.

Sodium nitroprusside is administered parenterally and is recommended only for short term use in intensive care.

Antiarrhythmic agents

The commonest arrhythmia in pregnancy, as in young people in general, is supraventricular tachycardia. It is important to exclude previously undetected disorders such as valvar heart disease, and even in an apparently healthy pregnancy the development of supraventricular tachycardia can occasionally be the first sign of pulmonary embolism. The occurrence of an arrhythmia in pregnancy requires assessment and management in hospital, preferably by doctors with experience in medical obstetrics. Antiarrhythmic prophylaxis is given for the same indications as in the non-pregnant state.

Adenosine given intravenously is used to restore sinus rhythm in paroxysmal supraventricular tachycardias when conventional non-pharmacological manoeuvres have failed. Adenosine is an endogenous nucleoside which transiently suppresses atrioventricular node conduction; it is safe to use in arrhythmias associated with accessory conduction pathways (Wolff-Parkinson-White syndrome, for example). Its rapid onset of action and extremely short half life support the expectation that the drug is safe in pregnancy, but experience of its use is limited. Individual reports of successful and apparently safe use of adenosine in pregnancy have appeared since 1991.[32–35.]

Amiodarone is an effective antiarrhythmic drug for the prophylaxis and control of tachyarrhythmias of either ventricular or supraventricular origin. The drug is not a first line antiarrhythmic even outside pregnancy because of its side effects. Amiodarone has a high iodine content, which can lead to thyroid dysfunction in the mother and potentially in the fetus. Other common side effects include reversible corneal microdeposits and photosensitivity. In the limited experience of the use of amiodarone in pregnancy, only transient neonatal hypothyroidism has been reported. The drug is reserved for severe dysrrhythmias resistant to other treatments. Amiodarone has also been used successfully to treat fetal tachyarrhythmia in utero, with resolution of hydrops and subsequent live birth.[36]

Digoxin is the drug of choice for the control of maternal atrial flutter or fibrillation. It is safe and effective, and there have been no reports of teratogenicity. Digoxin crosses the placenta freely, and toxicity in the mother can be fatal to the fetus. Renal clearance increases as gestation advances, so the monitoring of levels is advisable and dose increments may be required. Digoxin has also been used successfully to control supraventricular tachycardia in the fetus.[37]

Verapamil belongs to the family of calcium antagonist drugs but has a predominantly negative chronotropic action. Its use in pregnancy is controversial because of potential fetal bradycardia; this deserves mention because it is probably the most commonly prescribed drug in young patients for prophylaxis of paroxysmal supraventricular tachycardia. There have been no reports of teratogenicity, but verapamil has been used in only a few patients. Although verapamil has tocolytic activity in premature labour, it does not compare sufficiently favourably with traditional agents such as ritodrine for it to be adopted as an alternative.

Prevention of pre-eclampsia

Aspirin – It has long been known that platelets are involved in the pathogenesis of pre-eclampsia and several small studies suggested that aspirin could prevent pre-eclampsia in those at risk of the condition.[38] However, two large and well designed studies using 60 mg per day of aspirin have failed to confirm this early promise. In primigravid women aspirin reduced the occurrence of pre-eclampsia from 6·3% to 4·6% compared with placebo but placental abruption was increased sevenfold in the aspirin group, from 0·1% to 0·7%.[39] When studied in women in their second pregnancy who had experienced pre-eclampsia in their first, aspirin did not influence the occurrence of pre-eclampsia: 6·7% in the aspirin group and 7·6% in the placebo group. On the basis of these findings, aspirin cannot be recommended for the routine prevention of pre-eclampsia.[40]

Key points

- If the need for treatment with antihypertensive drugs antedates pregnancy the drug may need to be changed

- Angiotension converting enzyme inhibitors are contraindicated in pregnancy

- Methyldopa is a safe antihypertensive drug for use throughout pregnancy

- β Blockers are safe antihypertensive agents for use in the third trimester but can cause growth retardation if started before 28 weeks' gestation

---

- The commonest arrhythmia in pregnancy is supraventricular tachycardia

- Prophylactic treatment is given for the same indications as in the non-pregnant state

- Adenosine can be used to terminate supraventricular tachycardia and is safe in patients known to have an accessory conduction pathway

- Adenosine is theoretically safe in pregnancy because of its short half life, but experience is limited

- Digoxin is safe and effective, but toxic maternal levels can be fatal to the fetus

- Amiodarone is a third line choice for resistant dysrrhythmias because of its side effects

- Both digoxin and amiodarone administered to the mother have been used successfully to treat fetal tachyarrhythmias

1 Broughton Pipkin F, Turner SR, Symonds EM. Possible risk with captopril in pregnancy; some animal data. *Lancet* 1980; i: 1256.
2 Guignard JP, Burgener F, Calame A. Persistent anuria in a neonate: a side effect of captopril [abstract]? *Int J Paediatr Nephrol* 1981; 2: 133.
3 Rothberg AD, Lorenz R. Can captopril cause fetal and neonatal renal failure? *Paediatr Pharmacol* 1984; 4: 189–92.
4 Knott PD, Thorpe SS, Lamont CAR. Congenital renal dysgenesis, possibly due to captopril. *Lancet* 1989; i: 451.
5 Kreft-Jais C, Plouin PF, Tchobroutsky C, Boutry J. Angiotensin-converting enzyme inhibitors during pregnancy: a survey of 22 patients given captopril and 9 given enalapril. *Br J Obstet Gynaecol* 1988; 95: 420–2.
6 Martin RA, Jones KL, Mendoza A, Barr M Jr, Benirschke K. Effect of ACE inhibition on the fetal kidney: decreased renal blood flow. *Teratology* 1992; 46: 317–21.
7 Bhatt-Mehta V, Deluga KS. Fetal exposure to lisinopril: neonatal manifestations and management. *Pharmacotherapy* 1993; 13: 515–8.
8 Redman CWG, Beilin LJ, Bonnar J. Treatment of hypertension in pregnancy with methyldopa: blood pressure control and side effects. *Br J Obstet Gynaecol* 1977; 84: 419–26.
9 Jones HMR, Cummings AJ, Setchell KDR, Lawson AM. A study of the disposition of α-methyldopa in newborn infants following its administration to the mothers for the treatment of hypertension during pregnancy. *Br J Clin Pharmacol* 1979; 7: 433–40.
10 Whitelaw A. Maternal methyldopa treatment and neonatal blood pressure. *BMJ* 1981; 283: 471.
11 Ounsted M, Cockburn J, Moar VA, Redman CWG. Maternal hypertension with superimposed pre-eclampsia: effects on child development at $7\frac{1}{2}$ years. *Br J Obstet Gynaecol* 1983; 90: 644–9.
12 Rubin PC, Butters L, Clark DM, Reynolds B, Sumner DJ, Steedman D, et al. Placebo-controlled trial of atenolol in treatment of pregnancy-associated hypertension. *Lancet* 1983; i: 431–4.
13 Pickles CJ, Broughton Pipkin F, Symonds EM. A randomised placebo controlled trial of labetalol in the treatment of mild to moderate pregnancy induced hypertension. *Br J Obstet Gynaecol* 1992; 99: 964–8.
14 Rubin PC, Butters L, Clark D, Sumner D, Belfield A, Pledger D, et al. Obstetric aspects of the use in pregnancy-associated hypertension of the β-adrenoreceptor antagonist atenolol. *Am J Obstet Gynecol* 1984; 150: 389–92.

15 Butters L, Kennedy S, Rubin PC. Atenolol in essential hypertension during pregnancy. *BMJ* 1991; **301**: 587–9.

16 Reynolds B, Butters L, Evans J, Adams T, Rubin PC. First year of life after the use of atenolol in pregnancy associated hypertension. *Arch Dis Child* 1984; **59**: 1061–3.

17 Fidler JA, Smith V, Fayers P, de Swiet M. Randomised controlled comparative study of methyldopa and oxprenolol in treatment of hypertension in pregnancy. *BMJ* 1983; **286**: 1927–30.

18 Gallery EDM, Saunders DM, Hunyor SN, Gyory AZ. Randomised comparison of methyldopa and oxprenolol for treatment of hypertension in pregnancy. *BMJ* 1979; i: 1591–4.

19 Dubois D, Petitcolas J, Temperville B, Klepper A, Catherine PH. Treatment of hypertension in pregnancy with β-adrenoreceptor antagonists. *Br J Clin Pharmacol* 1982; **13** (suppl 2): 375–8S.

20 Williams ER, Morrissey JR. A comparison of acebutolol with methyldopa in the hypertensive pregnancy. *Pharmacotherapy* 1983; **3**: 487–91.

21 Symonds EM, Lamming GD, Jadoul F, Broughton Pipkin F. Clinical and biochemical aspects of the use of labetalol in the treatment of hypertension in pregnancy: comparison with methyldopa. In: Riley A, Symonds EM, eds. *The investigation of labetalol in the management of hypertension in pregnancy*. Amsterdam: Exerpta Medica, 1982: 62–76.

22 Walker JJ, Crooks A, Erwin L, Calder AA. Labetalol in pregnancy-induced hypertension: fetal and maternal effects. In: Riley A, Symonds EM, eds. *The investigation of labetalol in the management of hypertension in pregnancy*. Amsterdam: Exerpta Medica, 1982; 148–60.

23 Michael CA. Use of labetalol in the treatment of severe hypertension during pregnancy. *Br J Clin Pharmacol* 1979; **8** (suppl 1): 211–5S.

24 Childress CH, Katz VL. Nifedipine and its indications in obstetrics and gynecology. *Obstet Gynecol* 1994; **83**: 616–24.

25 Carbonne B, Jannet D, Touboul C, Khelifati Y, Milliez J. Nicardipine treatment of hypertension during pregnancy. *Obstet Gynecol* 1993; **81**: 908–14.

26 Allen J, Maigaard S, Forman A, Jacobsen P, Jespersen LT, Hansen KPB, et al. Acute effects of nitrendipine in pregnancy-induced hypertension. *Br J Obstet Gynaecol* 1987; **94**: 222–6.

27 Barton JR, Hiett AK, Conover WB. The use of nifedipine during the postpartum period in patients with severe preeclampsia. *Am J Obstet Gynaecol* 1990; **162**: 788–92.

28 Sibai BM, Abdella TN, Spinnato JA, Shower DC. Plasma volume findings in patients with mild pregnancy-induced hypertension. *Am J Obstet Gynecol* 1983; **147**: 16–20.

29 Collins R, Yusuf S, Peto R. Overview of randomised trials of diuretics in pregnancy. *BMJ* 1985; **290**: 17–23.

30 Lubbe WF, Hodge JV. Combined alpha and beta receptor antagonism with prasozin and oxprenolol in control of severe hypertension in pregnancy. *NZ Med J* 1981; **94**: 169–72.

31 Rubin PC, Butters L, Low RA, Reid JL. Clinical pharmacological studies with prasozin during pregnancy complicated by hypertension. *Br J Clin Pharmacol* 1983; **16**: 543–7.

32 Podolsky SM, Varon J. Adenosine use during pregnancy. *Ann Emerg Med* 1991; **20**: 1027–8.

33 Afridi I, Moise KJ Jr, Rokey R. Termination of supraventricular tachycardia with intravenous adenosine in a pregnant woman with Wolff-Parkinson-White syndrome. *Obstet Gynecol* 1992; **80**: 481–3.

34 Mason BA, Ricci-Goodman J, Koos BJ. Adenosine in the treatment of maternal paroxysmal supraventricular tachycardia. *Obstet Gynecol* 1992; **80**: 478–80.

35 Matfin G, Baylis P, Adams P. Maternal paroxysmal supraventricular tachycardia treated with adenosine. *Postgrad Med J* 1993; **69**: 661–2.

36 Rey E, Duperron L, Gauthier R, Lemay M, Grignon A, Lelorier J. Transplacental treatment of tachycardia-induced fetal heart failure with verapamil and amiodarone: a case report. *Am J Obstet Gynecol* 1985; **153**: 311–2.

37 Harrigan JT, Kangos JT, Sikka A, Spisso KR, Natarajan N, Rosenfield D, et al. Successful treatment of fetal congestive heart failure secondary to tachycardia. *N Engl J Med* 1981; **304**: 1527–9.

38 Rubin PC. Aspirin and pre-eclampsia. *Current Obstetrics and Gynaecology* 1994; **4**: 166–9.

39 Sibai B, Caritis S, Thom E, et al. Prevention of pre-eclampsia with low-dose aspirin in healthy, nulliparous pregnant women. *N Engl J Med* 1993; **329**: 1213–9.

40 CLASP Collaborative Group. CLASP: a randomised trial of low-dose aspirin for the prevention and treatment of pre-eclampsia among 9364 pregnant women. *Lancet* 1994; **343**: 619–29.

10 Anticoagulants

MICHAEL DE SWIET

Anticoagulant drugs are used in pregnancy to prevent and treat potentially life threatening disasters such as pulmonary embolus, cerebral embolus, and thrombosis of artificial heart valves; indeed, pulmonary embolus (with hypertension) is a leading cause of maternal mortality in the United Kingdom.[1] But used incorrectly anticoagulants have the potential to cause equally serious bleeding in the mother and fetus, and long term heparin treatment can also cause bone demineralisation. So the proper use of anticoagulants is a crucial part of modern obstetric practice. This chapter considers the use of anticoagulants both in venous thromboembolic disease and in patients with heart disease who are at risk of systemic thromboembolism.

Heparin

Heparin is an acid mucopolysaccharide with varying chain lengths of molecular weight between 4000 and 40 000 Daltons. Heparin has some thrombolytic action but in general it is used to prevent further blood clotting rather than lyse clots that are already present. The higher molecular weight heparins also inhibit platelet activity.

Recently the heterogeneous chain length preparations of heparin have been fractionated into those of low molecular weight. Low molecular weight heparin has a relatively greater anti-factor Xa effect than antithrombin effect. This, together with the lack of antiplatelet activity, may decrease the risk of bleeding while maintaining antithrombotic activity. Because of high polarity and lack of lipid solubility neither high nor low molecular weight heparin crosses the placenta[2,3] or is excreted in breast milk.

Warfarin

Warfarin is a form of coumarin that antagonises vitamin K. In general warfarin is confined to long term anticoagulation rather than acute management, and in pregnancy there is the additional problem that the drug crosses the placenta and can therefore affect the fetus. However, warfarin is not excreted in breast milk. Numerous other drugs interact with warfarin and can dangerously potentiate or reduce its effect.

Thrombolytic drugs

These drugs lyse clots by activating plasminogen to produce plasmin, which breaks down the cross links of fibrin within the thrombus. First generation agents streptokinase and urokinase have had limited use in pregnancy; newer and more fibrin specific agents such as alteplase and anistreplase have not been evaluated in pregnancy. Bleeding is the major complication.

Deep vein thrombosis and pulmonary embolism

After emergency resuscitation for pulmonary embolus, the treatment of both deep vein thrombosis and pulmonary embolus may be divided into an initial acute phase which lasts for up to a week and a subsequent chronic phase lasting for several months, where the aim of treatment is to prevent further incidents of thromboembolism.

Acute phase treatment

Heparin

Most cases of venous thromboembolism are treated initially with heparin. To prevent further clot formation, relatively high blood concentrations of heparin must be achieved. Although up to 40 000 units a day of heparin have been given subcutaneously, this is not usually practical because of bruising and irregular absorption, and the initial treatment should be with intravenous heparin: initially a 5000 unit bolus followed by 40 000 units a day (approximately 1600 units an hour) given by constant rate infusion pump, aiming to achieve a concentration of 0·6–1·0 units/ ml as assayed by the protamine sulphate neutralisation test or to double the activated partial thromboplastin time when compared with control.

The only side effect of heparin in the acute phase is bleeding; its preservative, cholorbutol, may cause hypotension.[4]

If it is necessary to reverse heparin therapy, merely stopping the intravenous infusion will usually be sufficient. Blood concentrations will be undetectable six hours after the infusion has stopped. If the situation is more urgent the patient can be given 1 mg protamine per 100 units of heparin. With a continuous infusion of heparin, twice the quantity of protamine should be given to neutralise the hourly dose. No more than 50 mg of protamine should be given in a 10 minute period, since protamine itself can cause bleeding.

Initial phase, high dose intravenous heparin therapy is continued for an arbitrary period of 3–7 days; the length of treatment depends on the severity of the initial episode of venous thromboembolism and whether there is any evidence of recurrence. Studies using intravenous heparin for only 5 days have been performed only in non-pregnant patients with deep vein thrombosis, not pulmonary embolus.[5]

Promising studies reported in non-pregnant patients have used fixed dose subcutaneous low molecular weight heparin in the initial phase of treatment.[6,7] Hull's study showed not only the obvious advantages of subcutaneous fixed dose versus adjusted dose intravenous therapy but also less bleeding in the acute phase and fewer recurrences.[6] A different low molecular weight heparin has been used for prophylaxis of thromboembolism,[8] but low molecular weight heparins have not yet been evaluated for treating thromboembolism in pregnancy. They could represent a major advance.

Thrombolysis

Pfeiffer claimed successful treatment of deep vein thrombosis in 12 pregnant patients with streptokinase given as a loading dose (250 000 units by intravenous infusion over 20 minutes) followed by an infusion of 160 000 units/hour for 4 hours, with subsequent alteration of the infusion rate depending on the plasma thrombin time.[9] Bell and Meek discount the necessity for adjusting the dosage schedule and recommend a maintenance therapy of 100 000 units/hour for 24–72 hours after the initial loading dose.[10] Although Pfeiffer suggests that very little streptokinase crosses the human placenta,[11] pregnancy is considered a minor contraindication to the use of thrombolytic drugs, and expected delivery within 10 days is a major contraindication.[12] Since thrombolytic drugs may precipitate premature labour by causing an increase in circulating plasminogen concentrations,[13] there is a risk that the relatively minor contraindication will become a major contraindication. Streptokinase may also cause relative uterine atony because of the interference of fibrin degradation products with uterine contraction.[14]

If it is necessary to reverse thrombolytic therapy in pregnancy, aprotinin, which is a large molecule and does not cross the placenta, should be used rather than aminocaproic acid. Apart from the 12 patients treated in pregnancy by Pfeiffer,[9] other studies are only case reports,[13–15] and therefore there is not sufficient experience to recommend the use of thrombolytic agents in pregnancy other than in exceptional circumstances such as life threatening pulmonary embolus.[16] In our experience, streptokinase seemed to be life saving in a patient who was moribund from pulmonary embolus in pregnancy, but the cost was severe bleeding from a normally sited placenta.

Chronic phase treatment

Warfarin

A definite, though low, incidence of teratogenesis is associated with the use of warfarin in the first trimester.[17–20] The most common syndrome is chondrodysplasia punctata, in which cartilage and bone formation is abnormal.[18,21] The asplenia syndrome[22] and diaphragmatic hernias have also been reported.[23] Since warfarin crosses the placenta, its use in late pregnancy (after 36 weeks' gestation) is associated with serious retroplacental and intracerebral fetal bleeding.[24]

The question has arisen as to whether oral anticoagulants should be used at all after the first trimester.[25] By causing repeated small intracerebral haemorrhages, warfarin may cause optic atrophy, microcephaly, and mental retardation.[26] Gross subdural haemorrhage may also occur in the fetus before 36 weeks' gestation.[27]

The teratogenic risks may not be so great as anecdotal reports would suggest. Chen et al studied the outcome of 22 pregnancies in which the mother had taken warfarin in the first trimester and

20 pregnancies in which warfarin had been taken between 13 and 36 weeks. Warfarin was being used in the management of artificial heart valves. Although the spontaneous abortion rate was high (36% in those taking warfarin) there were no cases of chondrodysplasia punctata or microcephaly.[28] We compared the infants of 20 patients who had taken warfarin in the second and third trimesters with those of well matched controls and found no difference in intellectual attainment at a mean age of 4 years.[29] Microcephaly is therefore unlikely to be common in the children of women taking warfarin. It may relate to the method of monitoring used for warfarin therapy and therefore to the amount of warfarin taken. Malformations of the central nervous system seem to be more common when the mother has taken higher doses of warfarin.

For the mother, bleeding also seems to be more of a problem with warfarin than with heparin, even if the prothrombin time is within the normal therapeutic range.[30] Fetomaternal haemorrhage has also been reported.[31]

For all these reasons conventional doses of warfarin should not be used in the chronic phase of treatment of venous thromboembolism in pregnancy or in the first week of the puerperium. Warfarin is recommended in pregnancy only for some patients with artificial heart valves or mitral valve disease (see below).

Patients may continue to breast feed[32] as there is no detectable secretion of warfarin in breast milk.[33] This is not so for phenindione: the breast fed infant of a mother given phenindione had severe haemorrhage.[34] However, phenindione may not be so teratogenic as warfarin,[35] but there are not sufficient data to confirm this.

Heparin

Subcutaneous, self administered heparin is the preferred chronic phase treatment for venous thromboembolism in pregnancy,[36] since it does not have the risks of warfarin. (The possible complications of long term treatment with heparin for thromboprophylaxis are described below.)

The half life of heparin injected subcutaneously is about 18 hours, whereas intravenous heparin has a half life of $1\frac{1}{2}$ hours. Most patients are given acute phase high dose intravenous heparin for 3–7 days (though some with massive deep vein thrombosis or severe pulmonary embolus may benefit from intravenous heparin for up to 14 days). They are then given subcutaneous heparin, initially 10 000 units twice daily. Provided there is detectable heparin activity, it is not usual to increase the dose of heparin above 10 000 units every 12 hours. If the concentration of heparin exceeds 0·2 unit/ml, the dose is reduced, since such concentrations are associated with excessive bleeding.[37] Heparin concentrations are stable in patients who are taking subcutaneous heparin, but because of pregnancy induced changes in blood volume and renal handling of heparin, and because treatment with heparin may continue for up to six months, heparin should be measured repeatedly, about as frequently as the patient attends for normal antenatal visits.

With the kits currently available, the activity of heparin against factor Xa has become easier to measure. An acceptable alternative is to measure the thrombin time as part of the normal clotting screen. The thrombin time is very sensitive to heparin, and patients who are taking more than prophylactic doses of heparin show a definite prolongation of the thrombin time. This allows the risk of bleeding to be assessed in patients taking subcutaneous heparin: if thrombin time is not prolonged, the patients will not bleed.

Because of the high incidence of thromboembolism in the days following labour and delivery,[38] subcutaneous heparin should be given through labour. The heparin concentration or thrombin time can be checked in the week before delivery is expected, since patients attend the hospital weekly at this time in pregnancy. There is no increased risk of intrapartum or postpartum haemorrhage,[39,40] except in those patients who inadvertently are taking too much heparin.[41] If thrombin time is normal, epidural block is now not contraindicated,[42] although it had been thought that there was an excessive risk of epidural haematoma.[43]

After delivery, the dose of subcutaneous heparin is empirically reduced to 7500 units twice daily because of the contraction in circulating blood volume and because the clotting factors return to normal levels during the puerperium. The heparin concentration should be checked at least once after delivery if the patient continues to take subcutaneous heparin for the recommended 6 weeks after delivery. Alternatively, 1 week after delivery, when the risk of secondary postpartum haemorrhage is much less, the patient may take warfarin rather than heparin. In either case breast feeding is safe. Neither warfarin nor heparin is excreted in breast milk; whether to continue heparin or to switch to warfarin depends on which the patient finds most convenient.

If heparin treatment is started in pregnancy or if warfarin is introduced more than 7 days after delivery, treatment should be continued for an arbitrary period of 6 weeks after delivery, at which time the extra risk of thromboembolism associated with pregnancy is considered to have passed. Patients who develop venous thromboembolism in the puerperium should be treated as above, except that after the acute phase warfarin may be used alone in chronic phase treatment if it is not given for the first 7 days after delivery. The total length of anticoagulant treatment should be 6 months.

Prophylaxis of thromboembolism

Prophylaxis might be considered in two groups of patients: those who are at high risk because of age, parity, obesity, or operative delivery,[38] and those who have had thromboembolism in the past.[44] With regard to the first group, it is generally believed (although not proved) that the risk of thromboembolism is greatest in the puerperium and therefore that prophylaxis need be used only during this period and in labour. The confidential maternal mortality series[1] clearly shows that the risks of thromboembolism increased greatly with increasing age. There is thus a case for using some form of prophylaxis, such as low dose heparin, in all patients who have had bed rest for at least one week before delivery; in obese patients; in those aged over 30 undergoing operative delivery; and in those over the age of 35 or in their fourth pregnancy (excluding abortion), even if they have a spontaneous vaginal delivery.[45] This suggestion has not been evaluated by clinical trial.

The second group of patients is those who have had thromboembolism in the past; they are considered to be at risk throughout pregnancy. In a recent survey of about 650 British obstetricians, 97% said they would use prophylactic anti-coagulants for patients with a history of recurrent thromboembolism and 81% for a patient with a single episode of thromboembolism in the past.[46] Thirtyfive per cent of British obstetricians would still use warfarin for venous thromboprophylaxis.[47] This now seems unacceptable because of the maternal and fetal complications of warfarin treatment. The alternative is to use subcutaneous heparin throughout pregnancy. However, since these patients are free of symptoms at the beginning of treatment and because the treatment is being used prophylactically, the safety of such therapy for mother and fetus must be established even more rigorously than for its use in the treatment of established venous thromboembolism.

Heparin

The most obvious maternal complication of treatment with heparin is bruising at the injection site. This can be reduced by good injection technique, but rarely is it eliminated. Although this is undoubtedly an inconvenience, and at times painful, most mothers tolerate a degree of bruising.

A further maternal complication of prolonged treatment with heparin is osteoporosis (heparin induced osteopenia).[48–50] Griffith et al reported that heparin induced osteopenia occurs only in patients receiving more than 15 000 units heparin a day for at least 6 months[51]; however, bone demineralisation has been reported after only 10 000 units of heparin a day were given in pregnancy for 19 weeks.[52] In one series of 184 women receiving heparin thromboprophylaxis in pregnancy, the incidence of symptomatic fractures was 2·2%.[53] The cause of the osteopenia is unknown. Since heparin induced osteopenia is much more common in pregnancy, it is likely that the enhanced bone turnover of pregnancy[54] and the fetal demand for calcium[55] are contributing factors. A follow up study of patients taking subcutaneous heparin suggests that even those patients who are symptom free may have some degree of bone demineralisation.[56] This is particularly worrying because of fears that the osteoporosis will progress further at the menopause. Fortunately, a follow up study from Sweden based on radiological assessment of the spine suggests that heparin induced osteopenia does regress once heparin treatment has been stopped.[57] Also Ginsberg et al, studying 61 patients 2 years after long term heparin treatment had been stopped, found no difference in bone density in comparison with controls.

Heparin may also cause thrombocytopenia[59] with subsequent bleeding[60] or thrombotic complications,[61,62] and alopecia and allergic reactions. Thrombocytopenia either presents acutely as a result of platelet aggregation or occurs 7-10 days after treatment starts because of an interaction between platelets, heparin, and a specific IgG autoantibody.[63,64] However, these additional complications are rare in pregnancy. The risk of heparin induced thrombocytopenia seems to be reduced, but not eliminated,[65,66] by the use of low molecular weight heparins.

Because of the maternal complications of prolonged treatment with subcutaneous heparin, heparin should not be used indiscriminately. Our present approach is to counsel patients about the relative risks of prophylaxis and recurrence of thromboembolism in the antenatal period.[67,68] Subcutaneous heparin is used throughout pregnancy only in those patients particularly at risk – those who have thromboembolism more than once in the past, who have inherited abnormalities of the clotting or thrombolytic systems such as antithrombin III deficiency, or who have the lupus-anticardiolipin syndrome and a single episode of thromboembolism in the past. Patients are also considered at high risk if they have had an episode of thromboembolism and if they also have a family history of thromboembolism in a first degree relative, which suggests that they have an undetected form of inherited thrombophilia. Subcutaneous heparin is also used in patients who are particularly concerned about the risk of repeated thromboembolism, and in low risk patients when they are most at risk, such as during admission to hospital for surgery or bed rest.

High risk patients who will take heparin throughout pregnancy start taking subcutaneous heparin 10 000 units 12 hourly, as described for chronic phase treatment of established thromboembolism in pregnancy; they are monitored haematologically in the same way, and the dose is reduced to 7500 units during labour. After delivery the patients receive subcutaneous heparin 7500 units 12 hourly for at least a week and either subcutaneous heparin or warfarin for a further 5 weeks, making a total of 6 weeks of treatment after delivery.

Patients who have only had a single episode of thromboembolism in the past, no matter what the associated circumstances, are considered at low risk of recurrence in pregnancy. These patients enter the above schedule during labour or at elective delivery. They are given subcutaneous heparin 7500 units 12 hourly and are then managed in the same way as the high risk patients.

Although this regimen for low risk patients is a compromise since it does not provide any cover during the antenatal period before labour, we have not observed any cases of antenatal or postnatal thromboembolism in over 60 patients treated in Queen Charlotte's Hospital in this way. They had all been treated for at least 6 weeks for an episode of deep vein thrombosis or pulmonary embolism before the index pregnancy. It therefore seems likely that the study of Badaraco and Vessey, which suggests a 12% risk of thromboembolism in patients who have had deep vein thrombosis or pulmonary embolism,[44] very much overestimates the risk of antenatal thromboembolism; the risk seems to be 2% or less.

In another study of thromboprophylaxis with adjusted dose heparin, Dahlman noted thromboembolic complications in 2·7% of 184 patients treated over a 10 year period with heparin 13 000–14 000 units a day for a mean of 17 weeks.[53] The failures were all in patients who had unsatisfactory levels of heparin or were later diagnosed to have a specific cause of thrombophilia such as antithrombin III deficiency; recurrence could probably have been prevented either by stricter heparin adjustment or by empirically using a higher dose of heparin.

Low molecular weight heparin

Low molecular weight heparin is used extensively for thromboprophylaxis in high risk surgery outside pregnancy – in orthopaedic patients or in cancer patients, for example. The advantages are once daily administration and possibly a better ratio of thromboprophylaxis to bleeding risk. At present cost is a major disadvantage.[69] We reported preliminary results of thromboprophylaxis with enoxaparin 40 mg daily in 16 patients,[8] and Gillis et al have reported results in a further 6 patients treated with enoxaparin in pregnancy.[70] Thromboprophylaxis was successful in all patients; those who had been using unfractionated heparin twice daily found the low molecular weight heparin less painful to inject.

Low molecular weight heparin causes significantly less platelet aggregation in pregnancy than does unfractionated heparin,[71] but heparin induced thrombocytopenia is rarely a problem in pregnancy. At present, patient acceptability due to the less painful once daily injections is the greatest argument in favour of using low molecular weight heparin.[72]

Low dose aspirin

Meta-analysis indicates that antiplatelet drugs reduce the risk of deep vein thrombosis and pulmonary embolus,[73] though no trials of low dose aspirin have been performed in pregnancy for thromboprophylaxis. There are extensive trials of low dose aspirin for the prevention of pre-eclampsia[74]; although efficacy for this indication is questionable, the safety record for both mother and fetus is good, the only risks being a possible slight increased incidence of accidental haemorrhage[75] (not confirmed in the largest study[74]) and in the need for blood transfusion.[74] We recommend low dose aspirin 75 mg a day throughout pregnancy for thromboprophylaxis in those at low risk of thromboembolism, as well as for high risk patients.

Anticoagulant therapy for patients with heart disease

Anticoagulation is a major problem in the management of patients with heart disease in pregnancy. It may be necessary in patients with congenital heart disease who have pulmonary hypertension due to pulmonary vascular disease, those who have artificial valve replacements, and those with atrial fibrillation.

Because subcutaneous heparin does not give adequate protection, warfarin should be used until about 37 weeks' gestation, even though the risk of fetal malformation such as optic atrophy may persist after the first trimester.[76] Furthermore, subcutaneous heparin treatment risks bone demineralisation. Use of the minimum dose of warfarin, maintaining an international normalised ratio no greater than 3, may well decrease the teratogenic and abortion risks of warfarin[77] without any increase in the risk of thromboembolism.[78]

At 37 weeks, when the risk of bleeding in the fetus receiving warfarin in association with labour seems to be too great, the patient should be admitted to hospital and given continuous intravenous heparin. The aim should be to achieve a heparin concentration of 0·6–1·0 units/ml as assayed by protamine sulphate neutralisation,[79] or to double the activated partial thromboplastin time when compared with control. It is believed that the clotting system of the fetus will return to normal after warfarin has been withheld for about a week. At that time, maternal heparin should be reduced to give a heparin concentration of less than 0·2 units/ml and labour should be induced. If the patient inadvertently goes into labour while taking warfarin, she should be given vitamin K to reverse the action of warfarin in the fetus and be given heparin as above. In extreme cases, vitamin K has been given intramuscularly to the fetus in utero by transamniotic injection.[80]

After delivery, because of the risk of maternal postpartum

haemorrhage, the patient should continue to receive heparin for about 7 days; then warfarin may be restarted. An alternative approach to anticoagulation in the early part of pregnancy was that of Iturbe-Alessio et al in Mexico.[81] They discontinued warfarin in 35 women as soon as they reported their pregnancy and substituted subcutaneous heparin 5000 units twice daily until the end of the 12th week, when they restarted warfarin, replacing it with heparin at the end of pregnancy. The results were compared with those in 37 women who continued warfarin throughout the early part of pregnancy. The control group had an extraordinarily high rate of embryopathy (30%), mostly diagnosed on the basis of minor abnormalities of the face. There were no cases of embryopathy and only two abortions in 23 women who discontinued warfarin before 7 weeks; there were two cases of embryopathy in eight continuing pregnancies where warfarin was discontinued between 7 and 12 weeks. The price to pay for this form of treatment was two massive valve thromboses in the group treated with heparin. Although the diagnosis of warfarin embryopathy must be questioned because of its very high incidence in the control group, embryopathy seems to be prevented by withholding warfarin between 7 and 12 weeks. However, a case of typical warfarin embryopathy has been reported in a woman who took warfarin from conception to 5 weeks and again from 12 to 33 weeks.[82] Ten thousand units of heparin per day is a very low dose in pregnancy and a more aggressive policy,[83] possibly with an adjusted dose continuous intravenous infusion,[84] might have reduced the incidence of embolism.

Conclusion

The use of anticoagulant drugs in pregnancy depends on the indication for the treatment. For established thromboembolism, heparin given intravenously and then subcutaneously is the preferred treatment for most patients. For thromboprophylaxis, high risk patients should receive subcutaneous heparin throughout pregnancy; low risk patients should receive antiplatelet drugs antenatally and subcutaneous heparin when in labour and for 6 weeks postnatally.

For patients with artifical heart valves, warfarin is the preferred treatment for most of the pregnancy. High dose intravenous heparin should be substituted well before delivery.

Key points

- Women with heart disease during pregnancy must be given adequate anticoagulants

- Warfarin causes embryopathy in the first trimester and can produce bleeding into the fetal brain later in pregnancy

- Osteopenia is an important side effect of heparin during pregnancy

- Women who have had a single venous thrombosis in the past could be given low dose aspirin unless there are reasons to consider that the risk is high

- Heparin prophylaxis throughout the antenatal period should be used in carefully selected cases: those with more than one thromboembolism in the past; inherited abnormality of clotting; antiphospholipid syndrome

- Heparin and warfarin can be used during breast feeding

1 Department of Health, Welsh Office, Scottish Office Home and Health Department, Department of Health and Social Security Northern Ireland. *Report on confidential enquiry into maternal deaths in England and Wales 1988–1990*. London: HMSO, 1994.

2 Hirsh J, Cade JF, O'Sullivan EF. Clinical experience with anticoagulant therapy during pregnancy. *BMJ* 1970; i: 270–3.

3 Melissari E, Parker CJ, Wilson NV, *et al*. Use of low molecular weight heparin in pregnancy. *Thrombo Haemost* 1992; **68**: 652–6.

4 Bowler GMR, Galloway DW, Meiklejohn BH, Macintyre CCA. Sharp fall in blood pressure after injection of heparin containing chlorbutol. *Lancet* 1986; i: 848–9.

5 Hull RD, Raskob GE, Rosenbloom D, Panju AA, *et al*. Heparin for 5 days as compared with 10 days in the initial treatment of proximal venous thrombosis. *N Engl J Med* 1990; **322**: 1260–4.

6 Hull RD, Raskob GE, Pineo GF, Green D, Trowbradge AA, Elliott CG, *et al*. Subcutaneous low-molecular-weight heparin compared with continuous intravenous heparin in the treatment of proximal-vein thrombosis. *N Engl J Med* 1992; **326**: 975–82.

7 Prandoni P, Lensing AWA, Buller HR, *et al*. Comparison of subcutaneous low-molecular-weight with intravenous standard heparin in proximal deep-vein thrombosis. *Lancet* 1992; **339**: 441–5.

8 Sturridge F, de Swiet M, Letsky E. The use of low molecular weight heparin for thromboprophylaxis in pregnancy. *Br J Obstet Gynaecol* 1994; **101**: 69–71.

9 Pfeiffer GW. The use of thrombolytic therapy in obstetrics and gynaecology. *Aust Ann Med* 1970; **19 (suppl 1)**: 28–31.

10 Bell WR, Meek AG. Guidelines for the use of thrombolytic agents. *N Engl J Med* 1979; **301**: 1266–70.

11 Pfeiffer GW. Distribution and placental transfer of 141I streptokinase. *Aust Ann Med*; **19 (suppl 1)**: 17–18.

12 National Institute of Health. Consensus conference thrombolytic therapy in treatment of pulmonary embolus. *BMJ* 1980; **280**: 1585–7.

13 Amias AG. Streptokinase, cerebral vascular disease – and triplets. *BMJ* 1977; i: 1414–5.

ANTICOAGULANTS

14 Hall RJC, Young C, Sutton GC, Cambell S. Treatment of acute massive pulmonary embolism by streptokinase during labour and delivery. *BMJ* 1972; iv: 647–9.
15 McTaggart DR, Engram TC. Massive pulmonary embolism during pregnancy treated with streptokinase. *Med J Aust* 1977; i: 18–20.
16 Flute PT. Thrombolytic therapy. *Br J Hosp Med* 1976; **16**: 135–42.
17 Abbott A Sibert JR, Weaver JB. Chondrodysplasia punctata and maternal warfarin treatment. *BMJ* 1977; i: 639–40.
18 Becker MH, Genieser NB, Feingold M. Chondrodysplasia punctata: is maternal warfarin therapy a factor? *Am J Dis Child* 1975; **129**: 356–7.
19 Kerber IJ, Warr OS III, Richardson C. Pregnancy in a patient with a prosthetic mitral valve associated with a fetal anomaly attributed to warfarin sodium. *JAMA* 1968; **203**: 223–5.
20 Pettifor JM, Benson R. Congenital malformations associated with the administration of oral anticoagulants during pregnancy. *J Pediatr* 1975; **86**: 459–62.
21 Shaul WL, Emery H, Hall JG. Chondrodysplasia punctata and maternal warfarin use during pregnancy. *Am J Dis Child* 1975; **129**: 360–2.
22 Cox DR, Martin L, Hall BD. Asplenia syndrome after fetal exposure to warfarin. *Lancet* 1977; ii: 1134.
23 O'Donnel D, Sevitz H, Seggie JL, Meyers AM, Botha JR, Myburgh JA. Pregnancy after renal transplantation. *Aust NZ J Med* 1985; **15**: 320–5.
24 Villasanta U. Thromboembolic disease in pregnancy. *Am J Obstet Gynecol* 1965; **93**: 142–60.
25 Venous thromboembolism and anticoagulants in pregnancy [editorial]. *BMJ* 1975; ii: 421–2.
26 Shaul WL, Hall JG. Multiple congenital anomalies associated with anticoagulants. *Am J Obstet Gynecol* 1977; **127**: 191–8.
27 Smith MF, Cameron MD. Warfarin as teratogen. *Lancet* 1979; i: 727.
28 Chen WWC, Chan CS, Lee PR, Wang RYR, Wong VCW. Pregnancy in patients with prosthetic heart valves: an experience with 45 pregnancies. *QJ Med* 1982; **51**: 358–65.
29 Chong MKB, Harvey D, de Swiet M. Follow-up study of children whose mothers were treated with warfarin during pregnancy. *Br J Obstet Gynaecol* 1984; **91**: 1070–3.
30 De Swiet M, Letsky E, Mellows H. Drug treatment and prophylaxis of thromboembolism in pregnancy. In: Lewis PJ, ed. *Therapeutic problems in pregnancy*. Lancaster: MTP Press, 1977: 81–9.
31 Li TC, Smith ARB, Duncan SLB. Feto-maternal haemorrhage complicating warfarin therapy during pregnancy. *J Obstet Gynaecol* 1990; **10**: 401–2.
32 Brambel CE, Hunter RE. Effect of dicoumarol on the nursing infant. *Am J Obstet Gynecol* 1950; **59**: 1153–9.
33 Orme MLE, Lewis PJ, de Swiet M, Serlin MJ, Sibeon R, Baty JD, et al. May mothers given warfarin breast-fed their infants? *BMJ* 1977; i: 1564–5.
34 Eckstein H, Jack B. Breast feeding and anticoagulant therapy. *Lancet* 1970; i: 672–3.
35 Oakley CM, Hawkins DF. Pregnancy in patients with prosthetic heart valves. *BMJ* 1983; **287**: 358.
36 Hirsh J. Heparin. *N Engl J Med* 1991; **324**: 1565–74.
37 Bonnar J. Thromboembolism in obstetric and gynaecological patients. In: Nicolaides AN ed. *Thromboembolism: aetiology, advances in prevention and management*. Lancaster: MTP Press, 1975: 311–34.
38 Department of Health and Social Security. *Report on confidential enquiries into maternal deaths in United Kingdom, 1975–1978*. London: HMSO; 1982.
39 De Swiet M, Fidler J, Howell R, Letsky E. Thromboembolism in pregnancy. In: Jewell DP, ed. *Advanced medicine*. London: Pitman Medical, 1981: 309–17.
40 Hill NCW, Hill JG, Sargent JM, Taylor CG, Bush PV. Effect of low dose heparin on blood loss at caesarean section. *BMJ* 1988; **296**: 1505–6.
41 Anderson DR, Ginsberg JS, Burrows R, Brill-Edwards P. Subcutaneous heparin therapy during pregnancy: a need for concern at the time of delivery. *Thrombo Haemost* 1991; **65**: 248–50.
42 Letsky EA. Haemostasis and epidural anaesthesia. *Int J Obstet Anesth* 1991; **1**: 51–4.
43 Crawford JS. *Principles and practice of obstetric anaesthesia*. 4th ed. Oxford: Blackwell Scientific, 1978; 182–3.
44 Badaracco MA, Vessey M. Recurrence of venous thromboembolism disease and use of oral contraceptives. *BMJ* 1974; i: 215–7.
45 Lowe GDO, Cooke T, Dewar EP, et al. Thromboembolic risk factors (THRIFT) risks of

and prophylaxis for venous thromboembolism in hospital patients. *BMJ* 1992; **305**: 567–74.

46 Greer IA, de Swiet M. Thrombosis prophylaxis in obstetrics and gynaecology. *Br J Obstet Gynaecol* 1993; **100**: 37–40.

47 De Swiet M, Bulpitt CJ, Lewis PJ. How obstetricians use anticoagulants in the prophylaxis of thromboembolism. *J Obstet Gynaecol* 1980; **1**: 29–32.

48 Avioli LV. Heparin-induced osteopenia: an appraisal. *Adv Exp Med Biol* 1975; **52**: 375–87.

49 Jaffe MD, Willis PW. Multiple fractures associated with long-term sodium heparin therapy. *JAMA* 1965; **193**: 152–4.

50 Squires JW, Pinch LW. Heparin induced spinal fractures. *JAMA* 1979; **241**: 2417–8.

51 Griffith GC, Nichols G, Asher JD, Hanagan B. Heparin osteoporosis. *JAMA* 1965; **193**: 91–4.

52 Griffiths HT, Liu DTY. Severe heparin osteoporosis in pregnancy. *Postgrad Med J* 1984; **60**: 424–5.

53 Dahlman TC. Osteoporotic fractures and the recurrence of thromboembolism during pregnancy and the puerperium in 184 women undergoing thromboprophylaxis with heparin. *Am J Obstet Gynecol* 1993; **168**: 1265–70.

54 Dahlman T, Sjoberg HE, Hellgren M, Bucht. Calcium homeostasis in pregnancy during long-term heparin treatment. *Br J Obstet Gynaecol* 1992; **99**: 412–6.

55 Misra R, Anderson DC. Providing the fetus with calcium. *BMJ* 1991; **300**: 1220–1.

56 De Swiet M, Dorrington Ward P, Fidler J, et al. Prolonged heparin therapy in pregnancy causes bone demineralisation (heparin induced-osteopenia). *Br J Obstet Gynaecol* 1983; **90**: 1129–34.

57 Dahlman T, Lindvall N, Hellgren M. Osteopenia in pregnancy during long-term heparin treatment: a radiological study post partum. *Br J Obstet Gynaecol* 1990; **97**: 221–8.

58 Ginsberg JS, Kowah Chuk G, Hirsh J, Britt-Edwards P, Burrows R, Coates G, et al. Heparin effect on bone density. *Thrombo Haemost* 1990; **64**: 286–9.

59 Hatjis CG. Heparin-induced thrombocytopenia in pregnancy. A case report. *J Reprod Med* 1984; **29**: 337–8.

60 Cines DB, Kaywin P, Bina M, Tomaski A, Schreiber AD. Heparin-associated thrombocytopenia. *N Engl J Med* 1980; **303**: 788–95.

61 Chong BH, Pitney WR, Castaldi PA. Heparin-induced thrombocytopenia: association of thrombotic complications with heparin-independent IgG antibody that induces thromboxane synthesis and platelet aggregation. *Lancet* 1982; ii: 1246–8.

62 Calhoun BC, Hesser JW. Heparin-associated antibody with pregnancy: disccusion of two cases. *Am J Obstet Gynecol* 1987; **156**: 964–6.

63 Cines DB, Tomaski A, Tannenbaum S. Immune endothelial-cell injury in heparin-associated thrombocytopenia. *N Engl J Med* 1987; **316**: 581–9.

64 Wolf H, Wick G. Antibodies interacting with, and corresponding binding site for heparin on human thrombocytes. *Lancet* 1986; ii: 222–3.

65 Eichinger S, Kyrle PA, Brenner B, Wagner B, Kapiotis S, Lechner K, et al. Thrombocytopenia associated with low-molecular-weight heparin. *Lancet* 1991; **337**: 1425–6.

66 LeCompte T, Luo SK, Stieltjes N, Lecrubier C, Samama MM. Thrombocytopenia associated with low-molecular-weight heparin. *Lancet* 1991; **338**: 1217.

67 Lao TT, de Swiet M, Letsky E, Walters BNJ. Prophylaxis of thromboembolism in pregnancy: an alternative. *Br J Obstet Gynaecol* 1985; **92**: 202–6.

68 Thromboembolic Risk Factors (THRIFT) Consensus Group. Risk of and prophylaxis for venous thromboembolism in hospital patients. *BMJ* 1992; **305**: 567–74.

69 Low-molecular-weight heparins in orthopaedic surgery. *Drug and Therapeutics Bulletin* 1993; **31**: 37–8.

70 Gillis S, Shushan A, Eldor A. Use of low molecular weight heparin for prophylaxis and treatment of thromboembolism in pregnancy. *Int J Gynecol Obstet* 1992; **39**: 297–301.

71 Ajayi AA, Horn EH, Cooper J, Rubin C. Effect of unfractionated heparin and the low molecular weight heparins, dalteparin and enoxparin on platelet behaviour in pregnancy. Proceedings of the BPS 1992.

72 Nelson-Piercy C. Low molecular weight heparin for obstetric thromboprophylaxis. *Br J Obstet Gynaecol* 1994; **101**: 6–8.

73 Antiplatelet Trialists' Collaboration. Collaborative overview of randomised trials of antiplatelet therapy - III. Reduction in venous thrombosis and pulmonary embolism by antiplatelet prophylaxis among surgical and medical patients. *BMJ* 1994; **308**: 235–46.

74 CLASP (Collaborative Low-dose Aspirin Study in Pregnancy) Collaborative Group.

CLASP: a randomised trial of low-dose aspirin for the prevention and treatment of pre-eclampsia among 9364 pregnant women. *Lancet* 1994; **343**: 619–29.

75 Sibai BM, Caritis SN, Thom E, Klebanoff M, McNellis D, Rocco L. *et al.* Prevention of pre-eclampsia with low-dose aspirin in healthy, nulliparous pregnant women. *N Engl J Med* 1993; **329**: 1213–8.

76 Sahul WL, Hall JG. Multiple congenital anomalies associated with oral anticoagulants. *Am J Obstet Gynecol* 1977; **127**: 191–8.

78 Javares T, Coto EC, Maiques V, Rincon A, Such M, Caffarena JM. Pregnancy after heart valve replacement. *Int J Cardiol* 1985; **5**: 731–9.

79 Saour JN, Sieck JO, Mamo LA, Gallus AS. Trial of different intensities of anticoagulation in patients with prosthetic heart valves. *N Engl J Med* 1990; **322**: 428–32.

80 Dacie J. *Practical haematology*. Edinburgh: Churchill Livingstone, 1975; 413–4.

81 Larsen JF, Jacobsen B, Holm HH, Pedersen JF, Mantoni M. Intrauterine injection of vitamin K before delivery during anticoagulant treatment of the mother. *Acta Obstet Gynecol Scand* 1978; **57**: 227–230.

82 Iturbe-Alessio I, Fonseca M, Mutchinik O, Santos MA, Zajartas A, Salazar E. Risks of anticoagulant therapy in pregnant women with artificial heart valves. *N Engl J Med* 1986; **315**: 1390–3.

83 De Vries TW, Van Der Veer E, Heijmans HSA. Warfarin embryopathy: patient, possibility, pathogenesis and prognosis. *Br J Obstet Gynaecol* 1993; **100**: 860–71.

84 Rabinovici J, Mani A, Barkai G, Hod H, Frenkel Y, Mashiach S. Long term ambulatory anticoagulation by constant subcutaneous heparin infusion in pregnancy. *Br J Obstet Gynaecol* 1987; **94**: 89–91.

85 Nelson DM, Stempel LE, Fabri PJ, Talbert M. Hickman catheter use in a pregnant patient requiring therapeutic heparin anticoagulation. *Am J Obstet Gynecol* 1984; **149**: 461–2.

11 Epilepsy and anticonvulsant drugs

GUY SAWLE

Few situations focus the mind as well as the discovery that a patient being treated for epilepsy has become pregnant. Below is a checklist of the topics I consider when I see such a patient, and how I try to address each point. Much of what has previously been written on this subject concerns treatment with barbiturate drugs. Outside of specialist epilepsy practice, very few women of childbearing age are now taking barbiturates, and these drugs will not be discussed further. Despite all that is written below, more than 90% of women with epilepsy have a normal pregnancy and deliver a healthy child.

Was the pregnancy intentional?

This is an anxiety about the use of enzyme inducing drugs in patients who are taking oral contraceptives. In practical terms, a patient who is taking carbamazepine or phenytoin needs "special" contraceptive advice, which generally means taking a higher dose pill. Usually 50 μg oestrogen is sufficient. If breakthrough bleeding occurs, contraception cannot be assured. An easy way to increase the oestrogen dose a little further is to take two 30 μg pills. Some patients need higher doses still, and it may be necessary to measure endogenous progesterone concentrations to confirm suppression of the luteal phase rise to be sure that ovulation is inhibited. Sodium valproate does not cause oral contraceptive failure.

Has the patient been taking folate supplements before conception?

One of the few things doctors can do that will most likely reduce the risk of fetal harm from anticonvulsants is to prescribe folate supplements in the period before conception. Folate concentrations in serum and red cells fall during pregnancy (more so in women taking anticonvulsant drugs[1]), and blood folate concentrations may have been lower in epileptic mothers who have an abnormal pregnancy outcome.[1] Neural tube defects are more common in patients taking valproate or carbamazepine (see below). Folate supplements are recommended for women who have previously given birth to a child with a neural tube defect,[2] and because of the association between anticonvulsant use and neural tube defects, it seems sensible to recommend folate supplements for all epileptic women of childbearing potential. A daily dose of 4 mg is the simplest and most convenient prescription, even though a lower dose would probably suffice. Because the timing of pregnancy is notoriously difficult to predict, the only practical way to ensure that women take folate supplements at the right time is to prescribe them immediately upon making a diagnosis of epilepsy during the childbearing years.

Does the patient really have epilepsy?

This should already be clearly known, but this is a good time to reconsider the evidence. Patients with panic attacks, cardiac dysrhythmias, and syncope are more likely to be harmed than helped by taking anticonvulsants during pregnancy.

Does the patient still need anticonvulsants?

Decisions about when to stop anticonvulsants are difficult. In general, if medication is stopped after several years free of seizures then the chance of that patient having further seizures rises to about 40% over the next few years. This sounds a high risk until it is appreciated that about 20% of a similar group of patients will have recurrent seizures over the next few years even if they continue to take their medication. Some diagnoses, such as juvenile myoclonic epilepsy,[3] carry a particularly high risk of seizures recurring after treatment has been stopped; here the neurologist's skills in diagnosis may facilitate appropriate management. Patients whose epilepsy has been difficult to control may be at greater risk of recurrence after stopping their medication. A decision on whether anticonvulsants should be stopped should thus be based in part on an understanding of the epileptic diagnosis and the treatment record to date. The driving regulations may also be relevant: patients with epilepsy are usually eligible to drive once they have been free of seizures for one year.

Once a woman knows she is pregnant the time of greatest potential teratogenic risk has probably passed, so being pregnant is not really a strong reason to stop taking anticonvulsants. If the drugs are to be stopped they should be withdrawn slowly, as they would be in a patient who was not pregnant. Recommendations vary about how quickly anticonvulsants should be withdrawn. It is normally best to stop in decrements over several months. In adults, each step should not exceed carbamazepine 200 mg, phenobarbitone 30 mg, phenytoin 50 mg, primidone 125 mg, and sodium valproate 200 mg.[4]

Is the patient taking the right anticonvulsant?

There is a tradition in contemporary neurological practice to prescribe carbamazepine for patients whose seizures are of focal origin (such as in temporal lobe epilepsy) and sodium valproate for patients who have primary generalised epilepsy (such as absence seizures or juvenile myoclonic epilepsy). With few exceptions both drugs are probably equally effective for either patient group.[5] A particular exception is juvenile myoclonic epilepsy, in which sodium valproate is the drug of choice and carbamazepine or phenytoin may make the patient worse.

A few years ago, carbamazepine was favoured for most women of childbearing age on the basis of a perceived lower risk of teratogenicity.[6] There have been reports of teratogenicity (including spina bifida) with carbamazepine, so switching almost exclusively to carbamazepine in women of childbearing potential would not now be regarded as expected practice.[7]

Some patients will be taking phenytoin. If seizures are well controlled and there are no side effects, there is little purpose in changing anticonvulsant during pregnancy, particularly as many of the putative teratogenic events will have already occurred before the mother realises she is pregnant (for example, the palate closes by the 47th day).

My patient is taking phenytoin, carbamazepine, or sodium valproate; what are the chances of teratogenicity?

This is the big question. There is an enormous literature on the teratogenic effects of anticonvulsants,[8] from which several conclusions can reasonably be drawn.

- Fetal abnormalities are more common in the children of epileptic mothers.[9] On the basis of the few published prospective studies of sufficient power to answer the question, it seems that there is an overall increase of about threefold in risk in patients with epilepsy (from about 2% in the general population to around 6% in mothers with epilepsy).[10] Most of this risk is probably due to the anticonvulsants rather than to the epilepsy itself.
- Abnormalities are more common when mother takes more than one anticonvulsant.
- There is a particular risk of neural tube anomalies when sodium valproate is used,[11] and to a lesser extent with carbamazepine.

Retrospective versus prospective studies

Many retrospective (and uncontrolled) studies have reported high rates of malformations and anomalies in babies of epileptic mothers. Unsurprisingly, prospective studies have generally reported very much lower rates.[12] Since the background rate of fetal abnormality is of the order of 1–2%, large numbers of both epileptic and non-epileptic mothers would be needed to have an 80% chance of detecting a doubling of this risk at $p < 0.05$. Few prospective studies have recruited such large numbers. In a large Australian study, nine malformations were recorded among 244 births to epileptic mothers (3·7%), in comparison with 2099 malformations amongst 62 265 babies born to mothers without epilepsy (3·4%). This represents a relative risk of only 1·1.[13] In another large (Norwegian) study, 170 malformations were recorded among 3879 births to mothers with epilepsy (4·4%), compared with 136 births to 3879 mothers without epilepsy (3·5%). In this case the relative risk was 1·25.[14] A more recent study with smaller numbers (119 pregnancies in mothers with epilepsy, 106 in mothers without epilepsy) concluded that there was an approximate doubling of the risks of an abnormal pregnancy outcome or minor malformation. In this case, the 95% confidence interval was also quoted (1·1 to 4·0 for "abnormal pregnancy outcome," 1·0 to 4·0 for minor malformation).[15] These figures underscore the need to view the results of small studies with caution, since even with over 100 women in each group and a finding of a doubling of the risk of an abnormal outcome, the confidence intervals almost include unity (that is, no increase in risk).

Fetal anticonvulsant syndrome

A host of congenital abnormalities have been reported in the children of mothers taking anticonvulsants, notably the "fetal hydantoin syndrome," described originally in babies born to five mothers, only one of whom was receiving phenytoin mono-therapy. This "syndrome" comprises microcephaly, growth retardation, and intellectual underfunctioning, together with a host of less serious abnormalities including ocular hypertelorism, distal digital hypoplasia, and craniofacial and other anomalies. Many of the dysmorphic features become less obvious as the children grow. Similar features have been reported in mothers treated with other anticonvulsant drugs,[16] and it has perhaps reasonably been suggested that the syndrome be renamed the fetal antiepileptic drug syndrome.

Cleft lip and palate

Cleft lip and palate are frequently cited associations with anticonvulsant drugs. A recent large case-control study reported an increase in the chance of non-syndromic cleft lip (with or without cleft palate) amounting to an odds ratio of 3·78 (95% confidence interval 1·65 to 7·88). In this study, both polytherapy and increased duration of epilepsy or anticonvulsant treatment increased the odds ratio. Nevertheless, in the group of patients studied (345 infants with either cleft lip or palate, 3029 unaffected infants), only 3.3% of the cleft lips and 0·9% of the cleft palates were thought to be attributable to anticonvulsant medication,[17] a reminder that congenital malformations and anomalies are common in normal pregnancy.

Spina bifida

The risk of spina bifida in children born to mothers taking valproate is of the order of 1–2%.[18] This is approximately the risk of recurrence in non-epileptic mothers who already have one affected child. There is also an increased risk in mothers taking carbamazepine.[19] In a meta-analysis of cohort studies published up to 1991, nine of 612 infants exposed to valproate monotherapy (1·3%) and nine of 984 exposed to carbamazepine monotherapy (0·9%) had spina bifida.[19]

It is particularly important that mothers taking sodium valproate or carbamazepine have α fetoprotein estimations and high resolution ultrasound examination at the appropriate time to detect neural tube defects. The combination of these two anticonvulsants may carry a particularly high risk in neural tube embryogenesis.

My patient is receiving polytherapy; is this really necessary?

Most patients with epilepsy are appropriately treated with a single agent. A minority require two or more drugs to establish and maintain satisfactory control of seizures. Women prescribed polytherapy for epilepsy during pregnancy have a very much higher risk of fetal malformation[20,21] (an unknown part of this increased risk may be genetic, since epilepsy that is difficult to control may itself be a manifestation of an inherited disease which is likely to lead to congenital abnormalities). The malformation rate escalated from 2·4% of 42 infants exposed to a single agent to 7·3% of 55 infants exposed to two agents, 16·7% of 36 infants exposed to three agents, and 25% of 16 infants exposed to four agents.[21] Few patients have been followed prospectively while taking particular combinations of anticonvulsants. In one such study, seven of 12 infants born to mothers taking the combination carbamazepine plus phenobarbitone plus valproate had congenital anomalies. One possible mechanism of increased teratogenicity with polytherapy may be that the 10,11 epoxide metabolite of carbamazepine (an active and teratogenic metabolite) is less well metabolised in the presence of other anticonvulsants.[21]

My patient is taking vigabatrin, lamotrigine, or gabapentin; what are the chances of teratogenicity?

There are very few data on the safety of these agents in human pregnancy. The potential teratogenic effects of newer agents should be discussed with women of childbearing age with severe epilepsy unresponsive to other agents, before these agents are prescribed. Since they are presently (1995) licensed as add on treatments, most patients who have received these agents during pregnancy have by definition been receiving polytherapy for epilepsy that has not otherwise been easy to treat.

Vigabatrin has been commercially available in western Europe since the end of 1989. The data sheet contraindicates the use of vigabatrin during pregnancy because of a lack of sufficient human data and an increase in cleft palate in rabbits when used at high doses (this may or may not be a teratogenic effect). Data collected by the manufacturers up to July 1994 include information from 55 pregnancies in women receiving vigabatrin in addition to other anticonvulsant drugs; these include spontaneous reports and active collection by the manufacturers contacting selected prescribing physicians. Various adverse outcomes have been reported (as expected in patients receiving polytherapy). In more than half of the cases, there has been a normal outcome.

Lamotrigine has been subjected to a wide range of mutagenicity tests in animals and the results of these tests have been interpreted to indicate that it does not present a genetic risk to humans. Nevertheless, it has been administered to only a few pregnant women and there are as yet insufficient data to properly evaluate its safety. Data up to May 1994 include 55 patients, of whom 53 were registered prospectively; in these 53, 34 live births were recorded with no birth defects noted. There were four spontaneous fetal losses, 13 induced abortions, and two birth defects (one case of spina bifida; pregnancy terminated at 19 weeks; mother also took sodium valproate; and one case of polydactyly; mother also took carbamazepine; previous child with multiple congenital anomalies).

Gabapentin has been shown to be neither genotoxic nor mutagenic by standard (animal) testing. Nevertheless, there are insufficient patient data to assess its safety during human pregnancy. Data collected by the manufacturers up to December 1994 include seven pregnancies. In all cases the mothers were also taking carbamazepine; some were also taking valproate, primidone, or phenobarbitone. Three pregnancies resulted in normal healthy infants. One mother delivered at 30 weeks; the child had respiratory distress syndrome but was normal at 13 months. The remaining three pregnancies were terminated by elective abortion.

Is there a genetic effect relevant to epilepsy and malformations?

There is a small literature regarding the effect of paternal epilepsy on fetal wellbeing. Most studies have found no excess of fetal abnormality in babies born to fathers with epilepsy.[22] In a study of congenital heart defects in 2461 live born children of parents with epilepsy the rate of malformation was similar whether mother or father had epilepsy (1093 mothers with epilepsy, 10 heart defects; 979 fathers, 8 heart defects), and the prevalence of congenital heart defects was similar to that in the background population.[23]

Will pregnancy affect the frequency of seizures?

Seizure frequency has been monitored in a small number of women with epilepsy who were not receiving anticonvulsants. In one such study of 23 pregnancies, seizure frequency increased in eight (35%).[24] Other authors reported very little (if any) significant change.[25,26] In women receiving anticonvulsants, most published data suggest that 30–50% have more seizures during pregnancy and 10–15% have fewer seizures than during preceding months. It may be that mothers who have fairly frequent seizures (outside of pregnancy) are more likely to have an increase in frequency of seizures during pregnancy than mothers who have very infrequent attacks.[27] Sleep disturbance or deprivation during pregnancy has been held to be an important factor in changing seizure frequency, and changes in compliance and pharmacokinetics are also likely to be relevant.

Will the mother have stopped or reduced her anticonvulsant dose?

Most expectant mothers are wary about taking any form of drug treatment during pregnancy. Given that many will think twice before taking simple analgesia for a headache, it comes as no surprise that women with epilepsy worry about taking anticonvulsants throughout pregnancy. The risk of taking drugs is seen as a balance between benefits to the mother and harm to the unborn child (perceived as possible mayhem). Mothers may feel they are being "selfish" if they continue to take tablets to prevent the manifestations of an apparently intermittent disorder such as epilepsy. Accordingly, an unknown number of women either stop taking or reduce the dose of previously prescribed drugs. In one Japanese study, 27% were considered to be poorly compliant and suffered increased numbers of seizures.[28] In a European study, 68% of the patients whose seizure frequency increased during pregnancy were reported to have been non-compliant.[24]

What about the effect of vomiting in pregnancy?

Tablets that are vomited after being swallowed are unlikely to provide good anticonvulsant effect. It is hard to know how vomiting affects the efficacy of anticonvulsant medication. It seems reasonable to suggest that patients should take a further dose if they recognise tablets in their vomit. Changing the time when tablets are taken may be helpful.

Is the patient taking the right dose; should I increase or decrease it?

Even with perfect compliance, serum concentrations of anticonvulsants are liable to fall during pregnancy as a consequence of changes in circulating blood volume, protein binding, and drug clearance.[29] The ratio of free to total anticonvulsant changes, mostly in favour of an increase in the proportion of free drug. The greatest change in carbamazepine concentration occurs during the third trimester, but for other agents changes may be more pronounced earlier in pregnancy.

In some mothers, increasingly frequent seizures during pregnancy may be the consequence of pharmacokinetic changes that lower cerebral concentrations of anticonvulsants, even though the dosing schedule previously controlled seizures adequately. Outside of pregnancy, patients with epilepsy who suffer further seizures are typically prescribed an increase in their anticonvulsant dose. Pregnant patients with epilepsy who have further seizures are appropriately treated in the same way. If side effects supervene after the pregnancy has finished, dosage should be decreased.

Outside of pregnancy, the best dose of an anticonvulsant is the dose that prevents seizures but does not lead to toxicity. Serum concentrations of some anticonvulsants (such as phenytoin and carbamazepine) may be used as a guide, but many (perhaps most) neurologists practising in the United Kingdom would use clinical, rather than laboratory, data to guide their prescribing.

Because of the known tendency for anticonvulsant concentrations to change in pregnancy and because of the known increase in seizures in some patients during pregnancy (but without knowledge of how many are due to changes in compliance), it has been argued that serum concentration of the drugs should be measured before (or very early during) pregnancy and then the dose should be adjusted during the pregnancy to maintain the serum concentration that was effective previously. The relation between free and bound drug changes during pregnancy, so it would be appropriate, if using such a strategy, to measure free drug concentrations.

There is no clear evidence that such a strategy provides better control of seizures than optimising drug treatment on clinical grounds alone; if patients had seizures during, say, the six months before pregnancy, then their anticonvulsant dosage should be adjusted (upwards). Informed opinion is therefore divided on whether levels should be monitored with pre-emptive dosage adjustment on the basis of falling concentrations even if the patient does not have seizures, or whether the dose should only be increased if a patient has a seizure.

The case for measuring carbamazepine concentrations

Though I believe that there is a reasonable relation between serum carbamazepine concentrations and clinical efficacy, like many other practising neurologists I rarely measure these concentrations in patients receiving only carbamazepine. It seems rational to measure carbamazepine concentrations during pregnancy, and this is accepted practice in a number of centres. There may be very little change in the concentration of free carbamazepine.[30] Because the absolute amount of the 10,11 epoxide (an important active metabolite) may stay unchanged[30] and the ratio of the epoxide to total carbamazepine may increase,[10] measuring *total* serum concentrations may give at best a crude indication of any relevant changes.

The case for measuring valproate concentrations

The manufacturer's data sheet for sodium valproate states that "the pharmacological (or therapeutic) effects of Epilim . . . may not be clearly correlated with the total or free (unbound) plasma valproic acid level." Outside of pregnancy, most neurologists would measure valproate only in adults with suspected poor compliance (in which case a level of zero would provide useful clinical information). In pregnancy, concentrations of free valproate may rise, even if total plasma concentrations fall, so that a patient whose total plasma concentration falls may develop pregnancy induced valproate toxicity.[31] Thus the anticipatory measurement of valproate concentrations, and particularly the practice of adjusting dosage in symptom free patients solely because the total plasma concentration has changed, is questionable.

The case for measuring phenytoin concentrations

In a patient whose epilepsy has proved refractory to treatment with carbamazepine and valproate or who has had unacceptable side effects with those agents, treatment with phenytoin may be appropriate. The pharmacokinetics of phenytoin are notoriously non-linear, and the case for measuring drug concentrations in pregnancy is stronger than for other agents.[26] (In fact, many of the earlier writings on the subject of seizure control during pregnancy were concerned chiefly with phenytoin.)

Will the epilepsy affect the pregnancy?

There have been rare reports of mothers having seizures during delivery, at a time when the fetal heart has been monitored. A generalised tonic-clonic ("grand mal") seizure may lead to a profound fetal bradycardia.[10,32] Fetal cerebral haemorrhage and death has been reported after a series of seizures during pregnancy.[33] This underscores the need for good seizure control during pregnancy in the interests of fetal well being. Rarely, (non-eclamptic) epilepsy occurs only during pregnancy and recurs with successive pregnancies.[27] Status epilepticus is a serious complication of epilepsy; it has a mortality of about 10% outside of pregnancy and is no less serious during pregnancy; death of the child and of the mother have both been reported. It should be treated along conventional lines.[34]

Should special precautions be taken during delivery?

Most mothers with epilepsy have a normal, uncomplicated delivery. In those taking enzyme inducing drugs, vitamin K dependent clotting factors may be affected. It has therefore been suggested that pregnant women taking enzyme inducing anti-convulsants should receive vitamin K_1 20 mg daily for a week before delivery. Since the exact date of delivery is seldom known in advance, it seems sensible to start vitamin K_1 a month before the expected delivery date.[35] If this regimen is missed, the mother can be given 10 mg K_1 parenterally during labour. Even so, fetal K_1 concentrations will still be low, and babies born to these mothers should be given vitamin K_1 immediately after delivery.[36]

Babies born to mothers taking benzodiazepines (or barbitu-rates) may suffer withdrawal symptoms after birth.

Is special advice required regarding breast feeding?

Although most anticonvulsants pass into breast milk, they do so in low concentrations and infants are likely to receive a lower daily dosage from breast feeding than they did in utero. Calculations of the largest amount of drug likely to be received by a breast fed infant expressed as a percentage of the lowest recommended daily therapeutic dose for an infant are below 5% for carbamazepine and phenytoin and under 3% for sodium valproate.[37]

What should I tell my pregnant epileptic patient?

Most of what the doctor should tell a pregnant epileptic patient should have already been covered in discussions before conception, when epilepsy is diagnosed or treated during a woman's reproductive years. Nevertheless, a number of points are worth reiteration during pregnancy.

- More than 90% of women with epilepsy have normal pregnancies and healthy infants.
- The risk of neural tube defects is increased by either sodium valproate (1–2%) or carbamazepine (0·5–1%); appropriately timed serum α fetoprotein estimates and high resolution ultrasound examination are critical.
- Anticonvulsants that are clinically indicated should be continued throughout pregnancy; seizures during pregnancy may be dangerous; it may even be necessary to increase the dose taken during pregnancy to maintain control of seizures.
- Folate supplements should be taken throughout the reproductive years.
- Vitamin K supplements may be necessary later in pregnancy.
- Carbamazepine, sodium valproate, and phenytoin can all be taken while breast feeding.

The prescribing physician should also carefully review the epileptic diagnosis and the need for ongoing treatment (seizure type, date of last seizure, ease of epileptic control, drug history, and driving status may all be important here). The need for polytherapy should be carefully considered, where appropriate. If the dosage of anticonvulsants is increased during pregnancy it may need to be reduced again during the puerperium.

Key points

- Enzyme-inducing anticonvulsants (carbamazepine and phenytoin, but not valproate) reduce the efficacy of standard dose (30 μg oestrogen) oral contraceptive pills; higher oestrogen doses are usually necessary

- All epileptic women of childbearing potential should receive folate supplements

- Once a woman knows she is pregnant the time of greatest potential teratogenic risk has probably passed

- If a patient's epilepsy is well controlled and there are no side effects, there is little point in changing anticonvulsant during pregnancy

- Many authorities recommend measuring anticonvulsant concentrations during pregnancy – some recommend adjusting dosage on the basis of falling concentrations, even in the absence of seizures; others favour an increase only if the patient has a seizure

continued overleaf

Key points *continued*

- Measuring total serum concentrations gives only a crude indication of any relevant changes

- Free valproate concentration may rise, even if the total plasma valproate concentration falls; neither correlates particularly well with seizure control

- Because of its non-linear pharmacokinetics, there is a stronger case for measuring phenytoin concentration

---

1 Dansky LV, Andermann E, Rosenblatt D, Sherwin AL, Andermann F. Anticonvulsants, folate levels, and pregnancy outcome: a prospective study. *Ann Neurol* 1987; **21**: 176–82.
2 Folic acid to prevent neural tube defects. *Drug Ther Bull* 1994; **32**: 31–2.
3 GrÜnewald RA, Panayiotopoulos CP. Juvenile myoclonic epilepsy. *Arch Neurol* 1993; **50**: 594–8.
4 Withdrawing antiepileptic drugs. *Drug Ther Bull* 1989; **27**: 29–31.
5 Turjanski N, Sawle GV, Platford ED, Weeks R, Lammertsma AA, Lees AJ, *et al.* PET studies of the presynaptic and postsynaptic dopaminergic system in Tourette's syndrome. *J Neurol Neurosurg Psychiatry* 1994; **57**: 688–92.
6 Saunders M. Epilepsy in women of childbearing age. *BMJ* 1989; **299**: 581.
7 Chadwick D. Epilepsy in women of childbearing age. *BMJ* 1989; **299**: 1163–4.
8 Yerby MS. Teratogenicity of antiepileptic drugs. In: Pedley TA, Meldrum BS, eds. *Recent advances in epilepsy 4*. Edinburgh: Churchill Livingstone, 1988: 93–107.
9 Delgado-Escueta A, Janz D. Consensus guidlines: preconception counselling management, and care of the pregnant women with epilepsy. *Neurology* 1992; **42 (suppl 5)**: 149–60.
10 Yerby MS. Problems and management of the pregnant women with epilepsy. *Epilepsia* 1987; **28 (suppl 3)**: S29–36.
11 Centers for Disease Control. Valproate: a new cause of birth defects – report from Italy and follow-up from France. *MMWR* 1983; **32**: 438–9.
12 Pearse SB,Rodríguez LAG, Hartwell C, Russell G. A pregnancy register of patients receiving carbamazepine in the UK. *Pharmacoepidemiology and Drug Safety* 1992; **1**: 321–5.
13 Stanley FJ, Prescott PK, Johnston R, Brooks B, Bower C. Congenital malformations in infants of mothers with diabetes and epilepsy in Western Australia, 1980–1982. *Med J Aust* 1985; **143**: 440–2.
14 Bjerkedal T. Outcome of pregnancy in women with epilepsy, Norway, 1967 to 1978: congenital malformations. In: Janz D, Dam M, Helge H, Richens A, Schmidt D, eds. *Epilepsy, pregnancy, and the child*. New York: Raven Press, 1982: 289–95.
15 Steeger-Theumissen RPM, Renier W, Borm CTF, Thomas CMG, Merkus HWWM, Op de Coul DAW, *et al.* Factors influencing the risk of abnormal pregnancy outcome in epileptic women: a multicentre prospective study. *Epilepsy Research* 1994; **18**: 261–9.
16 Jones KL, Lacro RV, Johnson KA, Adams J. Pattern of malformations in the children of women treated with carbamazepine during pregnancy. *N Engl J Med* 1989; **320**: 1661–6.
17 Abrishamchian AR, Khoury MJ, Calle EE. Ther contribution of maternal epilepsy and its treatment to the etiology of oral clefts: a population based case-control study. *Genetic Epidemiology* 1994; **11**: 343–51.
18 Lindout D, Schmidt D. In utero exposure to valproate and neural tube defects. *Lancet* 1986; ii: 1142.
19 Rosa FW. Spina bifida in infants of women treated with carbamazepine during pregnancy. *N Engl J Med* 1991; **324**: 674–7.
20 Lindhout D, Meinardi H, Barth PG. Hazards of fetal exposure to drug combinations. In: Janz D, Bossi L, Dam M, Helge H, Richens A, Schmidt D, eds. *Epilepsy, pregnancy, and the child*. New York: Raven Press, 1982; 275–81.
21 Lindhout D, Höppener RJEA, Meinardi H. Teratogenicity of antiepileptic drug combinations with special emphasis on epoxidation (of carbamazepine). *Epilepsia* 1984; **25**: 77–83.
22 Annegers JF, Hauser WA, Elveback LR, Anderson VE, Kurland LT. Seizure disorders in

offspring of parents with a history of seizures – a maternal-paternal difference? *Epilepsia* 1976; **17**: 1–9.

23 Friis ML, Hauge M. Congenital heart defects in live-born children of epileptic parents. *Arch Neurol* 1985; **42**: 374–6.

24 Schmidt D, Canger R, Avanzini G, Battino D, Cusi C, Beck-Mannagetta G. *et al.* Change of seizure frequency in pregnant epileptic women. *J Neurol Neurosurg Psychiatry* 1983; **46**: 751–5.

25 Gjerde IO, Strandjord RE, Ulstein M. The course of epilepsy during pregnancy: a study of 78 cases. *Acta Neurol Scand* 1988; **78**: 198–205.

26 Tomson T, Lindbom U, Ekqvist B, Sundqvist A. Epilepsy and pregnancy: a prospective study of seizure count in relation to free and total plasma concentration of carbamazepine and phenytoin. *Epilepsia* 1994; **35**: 122–30.

27 Knight AH, Rhind EG. Epilepsy and pregnancy: a study of 153 pregnancies in 59 patients. *Epilepsia* 1994; **16**: 1–66.

28 Otani K. Risk factorts for the increased seizure frequency during pregnancy and puerperium. *Psychiatric Neurologica Japonica* 1985; **39**: 33–41.

29 Eadie MJ, Lander CM, Tyrer JH. Plasma drug level monitoring in pregnancy. *Clin Pharmacokinetics* 1977; **2** 427–36.

30 Tomson T, Lindbom U, Ekqvist B, Sundqvist A. Disposition of carbamazepine and phenytoin in pregnancy. *Epilepsia* 1994; **35**: 131–5.

31 Yerby MS, Devinsky O. Epilepsy and pregnancy. In: Devinsky O, Feldmann E, Hainline B, eds. *Advances in neurology volume 64, Neurological complications of pregnancy*. New York: Raven Press, 1994; 45–63.

32 Teramo K, Hiilesmaa V, Bardy A, Saarikoski S. Fetal heart rate during a maternal grand mal epileptic seizure. *J Perinatal Med* 1979; **7**: 3–6.

33 Minkoff H, Scaffer RM, Delke I, Grunebaum AN. Diagnosis of interactanial haemorrhage in utero after a maternal seizure. *Obstet Gynecol* 1985; **65**: 22–4S.

34 Shorvon S. Tonic clonic status epilepticus. *J Neurol Neurosurg Psychiatry* 1993; **56**: 125–34.

35 Cornelissen M, Steegers-Theumissen R, Koklec L, Eshes T, Motohara K, Monvens L. Supplements of vitamin K in pregnant women receiving anticonvulsant therapy prevent neonatal vitamin K deficiency. *A J Obs Gynecol* 1993; **168**: 884–8.

36 Manderbrot L, Guillaumont M, LeClerq M, LeFrere JJ, Guzin D, Daffros F, *et al.* Placental transfer of vitamin K_1 and its implications in fetal haemostasis. *Thromb Haemost* 1988; **60**: 39–43.

37 O'Brien MD, Gilmour-White S. Epilepsy and pregnancy. *BMJ* 1993; **307**: 492–5.

12 Treatment of diabetes

N J A VAUGHAN

Diabetes is probably the most common disease that influences the outcome of pregnancy. Two to three women per thousand of reproductive age are known to have diabetes before conception, and a considerable proportion of pregnancies in otherwise normal women may be complicated by gestational diabetes. It is therefore hardly surprising that pregnancy was one of five key areas identified in the St Vincent declaration, a statement of attainable targets for the outcome of diabetes care to which European government health departments are signatories. Its recommendations provide the basis of an action programme for the substantial reduction of complications of diabetes.[1] For diabetes in pregnancy the objective is to "achieve pregnancy outcome in the diabetic woman that approximates that of the non-diabetic woman."

Pregnancy is a high risk state for both the diabetic woman and her fetus, and the importance of good metabolic control in pregnant women with diabetes is now undisputed. Complications such as macrosomia, neonatal hypoglycaemia, miscarriage, intrauterine death, and hydramnios, as well as increased perinatal mortality and neonatal morbidity, can largely be prevented by intensive efforts to achieve strict normoglycaemia. Many centres now report that perinatal mortality in the babies of women with insulin dependent diabetes approaches the rate in the normal population. In these women the usual complications of pregnancy such as infection, hydramnios, pre-eclampsia, and placental insufficiency may also occur more frequently, and some specific diabetic complications, particularly retinopathy, may develop or progress rapidly during gestation. Furthermore, the rate of major congenital malformations is at least 2–3 times higher than in babies born to non-diabetic mothers and this directly relates to metabolic control before conception.

The use of intensive home blood glucose monitoring, education about diabetes, and outpatient methods of fetal surveillance have been central to the improvement seen in the outcome of diabetic pregnancy over recent years. Great emphasis is placed on a multidisciplinary team approach, the team comprising diabetologist, obstetrician, diabetes nurse specialist, dietitian, neonatologist and, most importantly, the patient herself. As a consequence, admissions to hospital have been minimised and, wherever possible, uncomplicated pregnancies are allowed to go to term.

Perhaps the most important decision is the choice of insulin treatment both before and during pregnancy. This must be tailored to the individual. Each patient must have an insulin regimen with sufficient flexibility to maintain a normal blood glucose concentration (3–6 mmol/l) throughout the day and night, without serious hypoglycaemia, and which will also accommodate increasing insulin requirements as gestation progresses. This chapter outlines the management of diabetes for women with established insulin dependent diabetes as well as for those with gestational diabetes who require insulin. The identification and treatment of gestational diabetes is not discussed in detail as this is not without controversy and is well discussed elsewhere.[2-4]

Metabolic changes in normal and diabetic pregnancy

Essential to the management of diabetes in pregnancy is an understanding of the metabolic changes that occur in normal mothers. Plasma glucose concentrations remain remarkably constant, although slightly lower than in the non-pregnant state. This is despite increasing insulin resistance due to changes in the hormonal environment, including increases in oestrogen, progesterone, and human placental lactogen. Enhanced insulin secretion is able to compensate for these changes, but if functional islet cell reserve cannot meet these increased insulin requirements, gestational diabetes will develop. As about half of patients with gestational diabetes develop non-insulin dependent diabetes later in life it seems likely that they already have an intrinsic β cell defect.

Initially the metabolic adaptations of pregnancy are concerned with increased energy storage, and most of the early weight gain seen in pregnancy is the consequence of fat deposition. The substrate demands of the fetus gradually increase, and by the end of the second trimester these are substantial. As a result there is increasing loss of glucose to the fetus and accelerated maternal fat mobilisation, leading to modestly increased plasma concentrations of non-esterfied fatty acid and ketones. This is sometimes referred to as accelerated starvation.[5] In women with diabetes this preferential transfer of glucose to the fetus is particularly damaging to metabolic control unless there is an adequate compensatory increase in dietary carbohydrate.

The fetal β cell is not ordinarily stimulated by physiological changes of glucose, but when maternal diabetes is poorly regulated the fetus is exposed to much higher concentrations than usual. This increased metabolite delivery stimulates the fetal islet, causing hyperinsulinaemia and β cell hyperplasia. Facilitated diffusion of glucose across the placenta becomes saturated at about 11 mmol/l, so that the rate of transfer of glucose to the fetus does not increase when maternal blood glucose rises beyond this level. Thus, the beneficial effects of maternal blood glucose control are only seen below about 10 mmol/l. Improvement of control from "bad" to "average" will have little physiological effect on glucose transport and be of no benefit to fetal development and progress. Fetal hyperinsulinaemia directly leads to macrosomia; it may inhibit lung maturation and surfactant production, and enhanced β cell responsiveness following delivery may result in persistent hypoglycaemia.

Organising diabetic care in pregnancy

Care should be focused in units specialising in management of diabetic pregnancy and is best delivered by a multidisciplinary team comprising a diabetologist, obstetrician, diabetes nurse specialist, dietitian, neonatologist, and ophthalmologist. Patients should be seen regularly and frequently (at least fortnightly, with telephone contact in between, until 34 weeks, and then weekly) before, during, and after pregnancy. Joint clinics, with an obstetrician, diabetologist, and diabetes nurse specialist liaising closely, are the optimal arrangement. Those women developing gestational diabetes should receive the same level of care.

Preconception counselling

Pregnancies in diabetic women should be planned. All women of childbearing age with diabetes who envisage pregnancy should be counselled of the need for their diabetes to be under good control well before they make any attempts to conceive. Despite the dramatic reductions of many of the complications related to poor metabolic control, the incidence of congenital malformations in children of diabetic mothers remains two to three times greater than the incidence in the general population. Fatal anomalies and multiple malformations still occur more frequently than in the normal population. This has been shown to be directly related to the haemoglobin A_1 concentration at the time of conception (figure).[6] Organogenesis for all sites in which the congenital anomalies of children of diabetic mothers are most common is essentially complete within the first six weeks of gestation, before the mother may realise she is pregnant. Pregnancy should thus ideally be deferred until good metabolic control has been maintained for some time. Evidence of this would generally be taken as a glycosylated haemoglobin concentration in the normal

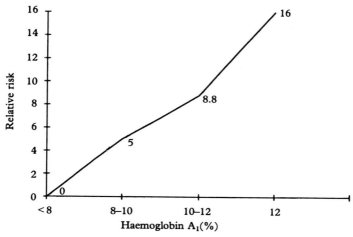

Figure 12.1   Congenital malformation related to 857 diabetic mothers' haemoglobin A_1 at conception[7]

range. Folate supplements should be started during this preconception phase.

Management of diabetes in pregnancy

Dietary prescription

Adequate dietary modification is perhaps the single most important aspect of management. Without this, achieving near normal control of glycaemia may be difficult or impossible. Dietary prescription must meet the needs of both mother and fetus, providing a total energy requirement of 30–35 Kcal/kg non-pregnant ideal body weight. Fewer calories than this will not allow efficient protein utilisation and may lead to ketogenesis induced by "accelerated starvation." Not less than 200 g (and preferably 220–240 g) carbohydrate should be consumed daily; this should comprise at least 45% of the total daily calorie intake and provide adequate fibre, calcium, and vitamins. This carbohydrate should be distributed throughout the day as regular meals and snacks, and it is especially important to provide a substantial bedtime snack (25 g carbohydrate and some protein). This helps to prevent starvation ketosis in the morning and to avoid nocturnal hypoglycaemia. Some mothers find that consuming this much carbohydrate is difficult, especially if nausea is troublesome in the first trimester. However, the dietitian plays an important role in finding acceptable solutions to this; often fruit and fruit juices, diet yoghurts, and even dried fruit and nut mixtures are useful alternatives. Protein requirements increase by about 30 g a day during pregnancy, and an intake of 1·3 g/kg is generally recommended, although many individuals already eat this much.

There is little or no place for calorie restriction in the control of diabetes in pregnancy. Nevertheless, in mild gestational diabetes it is usually worth attempting to correct a previously poor eating pattern, again by increasing complex carbohydrate. Good metabolic control can occasionally be achieved with such dietary measures, but such patients need careful observation with frequent checks on blood glucose and glycosylated haemoglobin concentrations. Deteriorating control requires insulin to be prescribed immediately; this would be indicated if the average of blood glucose concentrations before meals and 2 hours after meals throughout the day exceeds about 6 mmol/l.[7,8] There is no place for oral hypoglycaemic agents in pregnancy.

Insulin treatment

Several factors must be considered when selecting an insulin regimen. Nothing less than the attainment of normal blood glucose values throughout the day and night should be acceptable to either the patient or her doctor. Any regimen must be able to take account of the substantial changes in insulin sensitivity that may increase daily doses of insulin severalfold as pregnancy progresses. Regular home blood glucose measurements are essential to allow not only the day to day variations in blood glucose concentrations but also increasing insulin requirements to be met. Blood glucose should be measured with a reflectance meter with a memory (a useful check of compliance). With this degree of surveillance and the patient's almost invariably higher motivation, it is possible to achieve sufficiently good control with most insulin regimens that entail two or more injections of a mixture of insulins. There is, however, a trend towards using multiple injection regimens. It is probably best if radical changes in strategy are avoided, or at least started during pre-pregnancy counselling.

Choice of insulin regimens

It is preferable for pregnant diabetic women to use human insulin, although the few patients who are still using animal insulins, because of unawareness of hypoglycaemia, may be reluctant to change. Porcine insulin is probably acceptable, but bovine insulin is best avoided as it can produce insulin antibodies that freely cross the placenta.[9] These have been implicated as a cause of infant morbidity, possibly affecting β cell function of the fetus and influencing neonatal insulin secretion.

Once daily insulin regimens would seldom be appropriate in pregnant mothers with diabetes established before pregnancy, but single daily injections of an intermediate duration insulin before breakfast may be very effective in some women with mild gestational diabetes. Such patients can usually produce sufficient insulin in a fasting state overnight to maintain normoglycaemia and thus an intermediate insulin (an isophane such as Humulin I (Lilly) or Insulatard (Novo-Nordisk) or an insulin zinc suspension such as Monotard (Novo-Nordisk) or Humulin Zn (Lilly)) would be suitable. Additional short acting or soluble insulin such as Actrapid (Novo-Nordisk) or

Humulin S (Lilly) may be added later as a fast acting component to counter postprandial hyperglycaemia. Such regimens significantly reduce the incidence of fetal macrosomia in women with mild gestational diabetes in comparison with treatment by diet alone.[8]

Twice daily combinations of short and intermediate acting insulins – this regimen is widely used outside pregnancy and can provide adequate control during pregnancy as well. The usual combinations are a soluble insulin with either an isophane insulin or an insulin zinc suspension. Premixed formulations of these insulins should probably be avoided in pregnancy as they do not afford sufficient flexibility. Women using these formulations should change to free-mixing their insulins during the preconception period. The ability to change the proportion of short acting to intermediate acting insulin is important because as pregnancy progresses the required balance between the two may change with increasing insulin resistance. Hyperglycaemia before breakfast often cannot be resolved by increasing the evening dose of isophane insulin without incurring frequent hypoglycaemia during the night, partly as a result of increased transplacental passage of glucose. The general solution to this is to divide the evening injection, taking the short acting insulin with the evening meal and the intermediate insulin at bedtime. Similarly, as gestation progresses the proportion of short acting insulin required may increase, reflecting increased insulin resistance, and to control hyperglycaemia after the midday meal it is often necessary to abandon the morning dose of intermediate insulin in preference to an additional lunchtime injection of short acting insulin. From 36 weeks onwards there is a tendency for the fasting blood glucose concentration to fall, and this may require the evening injection of intermediate insulin to be reduced or omitted. Sudden dramatic falls in insulin requirements at this time should alert the clinicians to the possibility of placental insufficiency sufficient to threaten the pregnancy.

Multiple daily insulin injections are used by many younger diabetic patients who use pen-type insulin delivery devices. This is a particularly satisfactory means of achieving excellent metabolic control: it is readily understood by the patient and can easily be altered to cope with variations in diet and activity. Generally a soluble insulin is taken with each of the main meals of the day and an isophane or insulin zinc suspension at bedtime. Close self monitoring is essential for this type of regimen, but this will not differ from what is required in pregnancy.

Oral hypoglycaemic agents

The main anxiety about sulphonylureas in pregnancy is the possibility of further increasing the degree of fetal hyperinsulinaemia by direct, drug induced stimulation. Sulphonylureas cross the placenta and have been implicated as a direct cause of neonatal hypoglycaemia.[10] The long acting agent chlorpropamide is particularly dangerous and should not be used in the last 4 weeks of gestation. There is no firm evidence that these drugs are teratogenic.

Targets for monitoring of metabolic control

The mean diurnal blood glucose concentration in non-diabetic pregnant women is around 5 mmol/l at 30 weeks' gestation.[11] Diabetic women should be aiming at this level of control, attempting to obtain fasting and preprandial values of between 3 and 5 mmol/l and postprandial values of less than 10 mmol/l. Home blood glucose measurement is an essential aspect of management and should be performed 2–6 times a day to recognise the need for modifying the dose of insulin. This dosage adjustment can be performed by the medical team but the patient should be encouraged and helped to gain the confidence to undertake this herself. Concentrations of haemoglobin A_1 or haemoglobin A_{1c} should be measured regularly as this provides an objective assessment of glycaemic control. Target values should be the middle of the local normal range.

Management of labour

Dramatic changes in insulin sensitivity may occur in insulin dependent women at the time of delivery. Once active labour has started, insulin requirements fall. After delivery, once the placenta and its hormonal products have been removed there is a further rapid reduction in insulin requirement. Indeed, immediately after delivery insulin doses may fall below prepregnancy values.

During labour the simplest scheme is to use a constant infusion of 10% glucose at a rate of 1 litre every 8 hours. An independent insulin infusion of human soluble insulin, initially at 1 unit per hour, is also given; this is subsequently adjusted on the basis of hourly bedside measurements of blood glucose.[8] This system may be used irrespective of the last subcutaneous insulin dose, but where induction or caesarean section is planned it is best started at breakfast time after a bedtime injection of isophane insulin. As soon as the infant is delivered the insulin infusion must be reduced or, in women with gestational diabetes, stopped altogether. The glucose infusion should be continued until the next meal in patients who had vaginal deliveries or until a normal diet is resumed in those delivered by caesarean section. The prepregnancy insulin doses should be resumed at this time and adjusted according to the blood sugar levels. If breast feeding is planned, carbohydrate intake should remain at least 200 g daily. Patients should be warned about the risk of hypoglycaemia while feeding, especially in the middle of the night.

Although they are generally safe, care should be taken with the prolonged use of salt free solutions of glucose, particularly in conjunction with oxytocin (Syntocinon) and opiates, because hyponatraemia from water retention may occur.

Treatment of diabetic ketoacidosis

Pregnant women with diabetes are much more prone to diabetic ketoacidosis because of the combination of insulin resistance and accelerated catabolism of pregnancy. Initiating factors are the same as for any diabetic patient and include vomiting, infections, failure of insulin administration, or failure to meet increasing insulin requirements. Ketoacidosis in pregnancy must be treated with the utmost urgency as fetal loss occurs in almost 50% of cases. Patients are best managed on a medical intensive care unit along conventional lines but with close fetal monitoring. Adequate fluid and potassium replacement is essential in conjunction with intravenous insulin infusion, adjusted to achieve a smooth reduction of plasma glucose concentration. Initial rehydration should be with normal saline; this should be changed to 10% dextrose once the blood glucose concentration is less than 10 mmol/l and continued until the patient is free of ketones.

The use of corticosteroids in premature labour before 34 weeks' gestation to accelerate fetal lung maturation may dramatically increase insulin resistance. Similarly, the use of intravenous β sympathomimetic agents to treat premature uterine contractions will cause severe hyperglycaemia and ketoacidosis unless appropriately anticipated. Careful glucose monitoring should always accompany this form of treatment, and aggressive intravenous insulin treatment must be started if necessary.

Conclusions

In the past two decades remarkable improvements in the prognosis for pregnancy complicated by diabetes have been achieved. This has followed the recognition of the need for achieving near normal blood glucose concentrations not only during pregnancy but also in the preconception period. The multidisciplinary team approach is central to success. The choice of insulin regimen may at first seem bewilderingly diverse, but the number of injections a day that are used is important only in so far as it meets the patient's individual requirements to achieve normoglycaemia safely and without serious hypoglycaemia. No regimen is ideal; much depends upon the patient's cooperation and understanding. Complex regimens are not a substitute for education about diabetes and careful monitoring.

Key points

- The rate of major congenital abnormalities is directly related to metabolic control before conception

- All women of childbearing age who have diabetes should be counselled about the need for good control before conception

- Pregnancy should be deferred until glycosylated haemoglobin is in the normal range

- Oral hypoglycaemic agents have no place in pregnancy

- Corticosteroids or β sympathomimetic agents used in preterm labour will greatly increase insulin requirements

---

1 Krans HMJ, Porta M, Keen H, eds. *Diabetes care and research in Europe: the St Vincent Declaration action programme*. Geneva: WHO, 1992.
2 Naylor CD. Diagnosing gestational diabetes mellitus. Is the gold standard valid? *Diabetes Care* 1989; 12: 565–72.
3 Coustan DR. Gestational diabetes. *Diabetes Care* 1993; 16 (suppl 3): 8–15.
4 American Diabetes Association. Position statement: gestational diabetes mellitus. *Diabetes Care* 1986; 9: 430–1.
5 Freinkel N. Effects of the conceptus on maternal metabolism during pregnancy. In: Lerbal

BS, Wrenshall GA, eds. *On the nature and treatment of diabetes*. Amsterdam: Excerpta Medica, 1965: 679.

6 American College of Obstetricians and Gynaecologists. Management of diabetes mellitus in pregnancy. *ACOG Technical Bulletin* 1986; **92**: 1–5.

7 Stiete H, Stiete S, Petschaelis A, *et al*. Malformations in diabetic pregnancy. *Diabetologia* 1994; **37** (suppl 1): A172.

8 Gillmer MD, Holmes SM, Moore MP, Walters BNJ, Hockaday TD, Barringer BM. Diabetes in pregnancy. Obstetric management. In: Sutherland HW, Stowers JM, eds. *Carbohydrate metabolism in pregnancy and the newborn*. Edinburgh: Churchill Livingstone, 1984; 102–18.

9 Coustan DR, Imrah J. Prophylactic insulin treatment of gestational diabetes reduces the incidence of macrosomia, operative delivery and birth trauma. *Am J Obstet Gynecol* 1984; **150**: 836–42.

10 Adam PAJ, Schwartz R. Diagnosis and treatment: should oral hypoglycaemic agents be used in paediatric and pregnant patients? *Paediatrics* 1968; **42**: 819–23.

11 Gillmer MD, Beard RW, Brooke FM, Oakley NW. Carbohydrate metabolism in pregnancy. Part 1. Diurnal plasma glucose profile in normal and diabetic women. *BMJ* 1975; iii: 402–4.

Index